The Timing of Toxicological Studies to Support Clinical Trials

Discussion Meeting

The Timing of Toxicological Studies to Support Clinical Trials

Edited by

Christopher Parkinson, Neil McAuslane, Cyndy Lumley and Stuart Walker

Centre for Medicines Research
Carshalton, Surrey, UK

Proceedings of a CMR Discussion Meeting held at Nutfield Priory, Nutfield, UK, May 1994

SPRINGER-SCIENCE+BUSINESS MEDIA, B.V.

A catalogue record for this book is available from the British Library

ISBN 978-94-010-4623-7   ISBN 978-94-011-1424-0 (eBook)
DOI 10.1007/978-94-011-1424-0

Copyright

Contents

Preface

Over the past twelve years, the Centre for Medicines Research has held a series of Workshops on a number of topics related to the drug discovery and development process. The major objective of these Workshops has been to provide an international forum for regulatory, academic and industry representatives to debate together, and suggest solutions to, specific problems. The meeting reported in this volume represents a departure from this approach, in that the participants were drawn largely from the pharmaceutical industry. Senior clinicians, pharmacologists and toxicologists from companies in Europe, the USA and Japan met in May 1994 to discuss a scientific rationale for the conduct of toxicity studies to support the clinical development of new medicines, and to begin to work towards an industry consensus. Achievement of such a consensus is seen as an important step in the process leading towards international harmonisation of the recommendations on the timing of toxicity studies in relation to clinical trials.

In view of the fact that the 50 participants were drawn from 32 companies in nine countries, it is not surprising that there were many different points of view, resulting in lively debate. Three topics, representing the major differences between the current regulatory requirements in Europe, the USA and Japan, were selected for detailed discussion in syndicate groups: the minimum non-clinical package for initiating Phase I clinical trials; the duration of toxicity studies required to support repeated dosing in humans; and the timing of reproductive toxicity studies in relation to clinical trials. In the limited time available it was not possible to achieve a true consensus on all issues. However, the proposals presented by each group are published in order to stimulate further discussion in a wider arena and to illustrate the thinking of a small group of experts. The personal opinions of five toxicologists and clinicians on these topics are also recorded, together with chapters on international regulatory recommendations, current industry practices, expectations for toxicological investigations and the wider considerations for implementing a toxicity testing strategy.

The principal aim of toxicological studies on pharmaceuticals, using laboratory animals, is to identify the potential hazards in order to assess the risks associated with the administration of new medicines to man. The stepwise clinical development of medicines, comprising studies of increasing duration, patient numbers and diversity coupled with decreasing investigator control, necessitates a similar stepwise programme of toxicity studies for the assessment of the risks associated with the proposed treatment. Resolution of the anomalies between various guidelines on the timing of toxicity studies should serve to eliminate any redundant testing in animals and improve the efficiency of the drug development process by encouraging the use of single international strategies. As Dr Gwyn Morgan points out in his paper, this process of harmonisation should not be seen as a means of introducing less rigorous standards for the safety of medicines, but as a joint initiative by regulatory authorities and industry to rationalise the cost of drug development (in terms of money, resources and time) in order to increase the availability of new medicinal treatments to patients whilst also ensuring high standards of safety. It is hoped that this publication will provide important background information for the discussions on this topic which are currently taking place under the auspices of the International Conference on Harmonisation (ICH).

The Editors would like to thank all the Authors and Participants for making the meeting such a stimulating debate and special thanks go to the Rapporteurs and Chairmen of the discussion groups for pulling together the views into the consensus opinions documented in these proceedings. We are also indebted to Sandra Cox, whose work as administrator and compiler made a considerable contribution to the quality and timeliness of this publication, and to Jacquie Blanks for so capably handling all the administrative arrangements for the meeting.

Christopher Parkinson
Neil McAuslane
Cyndy Lumley
Stuart Walker

October 1994

Notes on contributors

John C Alexander MD was appointed Executive Vice President, Medical Research of Searle in 1991. He is responsible for all worldwide clinical development of Searle Research and Development compounds Phase I–IV and serves as the primary R&D medical spokesperson with the FDA and other regulatory agencies. Dr Alexander began his career with the Squibb Corporation in 1976 and progressed through various positions within the Clinical Research function and in 1990 he became Vice President Cardiovascular Clinical Research and Development for the new Bristol–Myers Squibb Company. During this time, Dr Alexander played a central role in the development of several important products including captopril and pravastatin. He is author and co-author of numerous publications and is also a member of the American Heart Association, Council on Epidemiology and Hypertension, the Society for Clinical Trials and the American Society for Hypertension.

Philip Bentley BSc PhD is Head of Preclinical Safety of Ciba Pharmaceuticals Division, Basel. He joined Ciba-Geigy in 1979 to research into mechanisms of toxicity and hepatocarcinogenicity, moved to the Pharmaceuticals Division in 1990 as Head of Drug Metabolism and a year later took his present position. He has published in the areas of enzymology, mutagenicity, drug metabolism and mechanisms of tumour induction by non-genotoxic agents. Dr Bentley is an active member of several scientific associations and is a past president of the European Society of Biochemical Pharmacology.

Professor Fritz R Bühler MD is Director of International Clinical Research, F Hoffmann-La Roche Limited. He is a professor of Pathophysiology as well as in Medicine and Cardiology and is the former Director of the Department of Research of the University Hospitals, Basel, Switzerland, where he is currently a consultant in Cardiology and Hypertension at the Division of Cardiology, Department of Medicine. Between 1970 and 1973 Professor Bühler worked at Columbia University in New York and in 1977 as a visiting professor at Harvard Medicine School in Boston. Professor Bühler is a member of several societies in the field of cardiovascular research, and he is an Executive Member of the Swiss Academy of Medical Sciences. As well as directing his main research interests in cardiovascular disease and editing supplements of the Journal of Cardiovascular Pharmacology, Professor Bühler was the Executive Chairman of the International Prospective Primary Prevention Study in Hypertension.

Professor Donald S Davies BSc PhD FRSC MRCPath is Professor of Biochemical Pharmacology and Director of the Department of Clinical Pharmacology at the Royal Postgraduate Medical School, University of London. His research interests are in mechanisms of drug action and toxicity and he takes an active interest in all aspects of drug safety and regulation. Professor Davies has published over 150 papers in peer-reviewed journals, has contributed chapters to numerous text books and has organised international congresses on toxicology. He is a member of the Committee on Safety of Medicines in the UK.

Jack H Dean PhD was appointed President, Sanofi Research Division, Sanofi Winthrop Inc, in October 1994, having joined Sterling in 1988 as Director of the Department of Toxicology. Dr Dean served as Director of the Sterling Winthrop Pharmaceuticals Research Division UK Research Centre from 1990 to 1992, and as Executive Vice President, Development for the Sterling Winthrop Pharmaceuticals Research Division from 1992 to 1994. Prior to joining Sterling, he headed the Immunotoxicology Section at the National Institute of Environmental Health Sciences and National Toxicology Program, National Institutes of Health. Dr Dean has been Adjunct Professor at the University of North Carolina, and at Duke University, Department of Pathology. He has served on the Executive Council of the Society of Toxicology, he is currently Vice-President of the Society, and the International Society of Immunopharmacology. Dr Dean is a member of the Pharmaceutical Research and Manufacturers of America's (PhRMA) Drug Safety Section Steering Committee. He also has served as a consultant to various review committees for the National Institutes of Health, the Centers for Disease Control, Environmental Protection Agency, the Congressional Office of Technology Assessment, and the World Health Organization. Dr Dean's research interests include the immunotoxicity of drugs and models for defining toxicity at a cellular and molecular level. He has edited four books and published more than 200 journal articles.

Alan Dunton MD was appointed Vice President Clinical Research & Development, Janssen Research Foundation, US in September 1994. Formerly, he was Vice President and Director, Center for Clinical Pharmacology and Pharmacokinetics, Syntex (USA) Inc.

Toshiji Igarashi BSc PhD joined Eisai Company Limited in 1959 as a pharmacologist in R&D. He became Director of New Drug Discovery Research in 1985, Director of Drug Safety Research in 1987 and he is currently Director, R&D Documentation and Information Technology. Dr Igarashi is Chairman of the Non-clinical Evaluation Committee of the JPMA and served on the Safety Expert Working Groups for the ICH discussions on the duration of repeated dose toxicity studies (Brussels, 1991) and toxicokinetics (Orlando, 1993). He is also a Senior Member of the Japanese Pharmacology Society and a Director Member of the Japanese Society of Toxicology Sciences.

Michael R Jackson BVM&S MRCVS PhD MRCPath is Director of Medicines Safety Evaluation at Glaxo Research and Development Limited, UK. He gained his PhD on rodent hepatocarcinogenesis from Edinburgh University after general training in laboratory animal pathology. Dr Jackson commenced his career in the pharmaceutical industry as a pathologist at Allen & Hanburys Limited and then broadened his overall interest in safety evaluation as Head of Drug Safety Department at Roche Products Limited. His continuing career at Glaxo has enabled him to pursue directing non-clinical safety evaluation of novel medicines. He is the immediate past chairman of the British Toxicology Society.

Professor Trevor M Jones BPharm PhD FPS CChem FRSC FKC MCPP was appointed Director General of The Association of the British Pharmaceutical Industry in August 1994. Prior to that he was Director of Research, Development and Medical, The Wellcome Foundation Limited with responsibility for all R&D activities worldwide outside the USA, and a Main Board Director. Some time Visiting Professor at the University of North Carolina and the University of Strathclyde, he is currently a member of Council and Visiting Professor at King's College, London University. He has been a member of the Medicines Commission (UK Government Department of Health) for twelve years and advises the Cabinet Office on matters relating to the Human Genome Project. He is also an expert on the Task Force on the use of Human Tissues: Nuffield Bioethics Council. Professor Jones is a member of a number of editorial boards and has authored numerous publications throughout his career.

Diane K Jorkasky MD FACP joined SmithKline Beecham in 1988 and is currently Vice President & Director of Clinical Pharmacology, North America. In her early career she specialised in nephrology which led to the position of Transplantation Nephrologist at the Hospital of the University of Pennsylvania. She holds the position of Chief of the Renal Metabolic Section at the Presbyterian Medical Center, an affiliate of the University of Pennsylvania. Dr Jorkasky is also Clinical Associate Professor of Medicine at the University of Pennsylvania, still pursuing an active teaching role for which she has received many awards. She serves on several of the University committees, is a member of numerous medical or pharmacological societies, and sits on the editorial board of *Annals of Internal Medicine*. Dr Jorkasky is board certified in medicine, nephrology, and clinical pharmacology.

Cyndy E Lumley BSc PhD is Associate Director at the Centre for Medicines Research, where she has worked for the past eleven years. Prior to joining the CMR, she obtained a BSc (hons) in Medical Biochemistry from the University of Surrey and a PhD in Radiation Biology from the University of London. Dr Lumley's current research interests include safety testing of new medicines, drug regulations, the predictive value of animal studies for man, pharmaceutical research and development expenditure, and factors affecting drug development. She is a member of the British Toxicology Society Executive Committee and of the editorial board of TEN. Dr Lumley is a regular contributor to scientific journals and international meetings, has co-authored over 30 research papers and edited three books.

Jeanne M Manson PhD is a Distinguished Senior Investigator at Merck Research Laboratories, Philadelphia, USA. She was formerly an Associate Professor of Environmental Health and Obstetrics/Gynaecology at the University of Cincinnati and has been involved in research and drug safety evaluation in reproductive toxicology for the past 18 years.

Neil McAuslane BSc MSc PhD is Project Manager at the Centre for Medicines Research, with responsibility for the safety evaluation/regulations programme. He has degrees in Pharmacology and Toxicology, and joined the Centre to initiate the control animal pathology database project. Dr McAuslane's current research interests are in the area of safety testing of pharmaceuticals, and the CMR's continuing study into the evaluation of inter-ethnic differences. He has edited three books and co-authored several of the Centre's publications in these research areas.

R Michael McClain PhD is Director of Toxicology/Research Advisor for Hoffmann-La Roche Inc, USA. Dr McClain joined Roche in 1970 and has held various positions involved in reproductive toxicology, general toxicology and carcinogenicity testing. His research activities include mechanisms of chemical carcinogenesis for thyroid, adrenal and liver, and regulatory aspects for cancer risk assessment. Dr McClain has been active in PhRMA for Drug Safety, the Society of Toxicology and ILSI.

Gwyn Morgan BVSc PhD MRCVS is Vice President of Safety Assessment in the Research and Development Division of SmithKline Beecham Pharmaceuticals, and formerly was a lecturer in Veterinary Comparative Pathology at the Medical School, University of Bristol, England. His research interests have included oncogenic herpes viruses, mechanisms of toxicity and pathogenesis of drug-induced arterial toxicity, and he has more than 50 publications on these topics. Dr Morgan is Vice Chairman of the US Pharmaceutical Research and Manufacturers of America Drug Safety Subsection Steering Committee and is a member of the Executive Council of the American Society of Toxicologic Pathologists.

Douglas M Morton BPharm PhD CChem MRSC MRPS is Vice President of Lilly Research Laboratories, a division of Eli Lilly and Company. He was born in the United Kingdom and qualified as a pharmacist at the University of London in 1963. After obtaining a PhD in pharmaceutical chemistry, he held an international post-doctoral fellowship at the US National Institutes of Health, Bethesda, Maryland, USA, in1966–67. Following his return to England, Dr Morton began his career within the Eli Lilly International Corporation where he held various positions before transferring to corporate headquarters in Indianapolis in 1974 as Director of Toxicology for Lilly Research Laboratories. Dr Morton was appointed Professor of Pharmacology and Toxicology at the Indiana University School of Medicine in January 1979.

Christopher Parkinson BSc PhD is Senior Research Associate at the Centre for Medicines Research, with responsibility for the research projects carried out in the regulations area. Prior to joining the Centre in 1990, Dr Parkinson gained four years' experience in the pharmaceutical and contract research industries as well as obtaining his PhD in Toxicology from the University of Kingston. His main area of research interest lies in the scientific justification of non-clinical regulatory requirements for pharmaceuticals.

M David C Scales PhD FRCPath FIBiol is Director of Toxicological Sciences for Glaxo Group Research, having responsibility for both Toxicology and Pathology Departments. After graduating with a BSc and PhD from the University of London and an MSc from the Royal Postgraduate Medical School, he trained as a Toxicological Pathologist with ICI's Central Toxicology Laboratory and gained membership to the Royal College of Pathologists in 1982. David Scales is Chairman of the ABPI Toxicology Sub-Committee, Chairman of the Centre for Medicines Research

International Safety Evaluation Advisory Board, and European Industry Representative on the International Conference for Harmonisation Expert Working Group in Safety. He is also a member of the Royal College of Pathologists Special Advisory Committee in Toxicology and the Specialist Advisor in Postgraduate Education to the Royal College of Pathologists. David Scales holds a visiting chair in Toxicology at the School of Pharmacy, University of London.

Kurt E Suter PhD is Head of Project Group in the Toxicology Department of Drug Safety, Sandoz, Basle, and represents the Department in various project teams for the development of pharmaceuticals in CNS indications. Dr Suter joined Sandoz Pharma Limited in 1975. Before his present position he was Head of Reproductive Toxicology and Regulatory Toxicology. Dr Suter has a broad interest in safety aspects of drugs and their regulations.

Toshimi Usui DVM PhD is Senior General Manager for Non-Clinical Safety Assessment in the Research and Development Division of Janssen-Kyowa Company Limited, Japan. He is a Vice-Chairman of the Non-Clinical Evaluation Sub-Committee, the Pharmaceutical Evaluation Committee of JPMA, and diplomate and council member of the Japanese Society for Toxicologic Pathologists, the Japanese Society for Veterinary Pathologists, and the Japanese Society of Toxicology. He is also a member of the European Society of Toxicology.

Herman Van Cauteren DVM is the Vice-President for Non-Clinical Safety Assessment at Janssen Pharmaceutica, Belgium. In this position he is responsible for the final toxicology of all new drugs of the Janssen Research Foundation worldwide. Prior to this Dr Van Cauteren was Director of Toxicology in the same company. In former positions he was a Research Assistant in the Department of Veterinary Medicine of the University of Wisconsin, Madison, USA, for postdoctoral specialisation in toxicology, pathology and cancer. He also was a Researcher in the Department of Internal Veterinary Medicine of the University of Ghent, Belgium. Dr Van Cauteren's publications mainly include papers on toxicology and drug safety. He also has been acting as the main author for several expert reports on the pharmacological toxicological documentation of new drugs.

Professor Stuart R Walker BSc PhD CChem FRSC CBiol FIBiol is the Director of the Centre for Medicines Research in the UK and Honorary Professor of Pharmaceutical Medicine, University of Wales, Cardiff. He spent ten years at London University which included lectureships in biochemical pharmacology at St Mary's Hospital Medical School and in clinical pharmacology at the Cardiothoracic Institute in London. This was followed by eight years with Glaxo Group Research in the UK where he had international responsibility for several of their clinical research programmes. His current research interests include studies into the process of innovation in drug research and development, an examination of the impact of international medicines regulations and policy issues on drug development, investigating the role as well as the predictive value of preclinical animal toxicology and measuring the socioeconomic benefit of medicines in therapeutic intervention studies. Professor Walker is a member of several academic, professional and industrial committees and sits on the editorial boards of three scientific journals. He is frequently involved in the organisation of national and international meetings on key issues that concern the pharmaceutical industry, and he has lectured extensively throughout Europe, Japan and the USA. Professor Walker has co-authored over 150 research papers and edited fourteen books.

Robert L Zerbe MD is Senior Vice-President, Worldwide Clinical Investigation, Parke-Davis Pharmaceutical Research. Dr Zerbe graduated from Indiana University, where he also served his internship, residency and a fellowship. He was a Senior Staff Fellow at the National Institute of Mental Health prior to joining Lilly in June 1982 as an associate clinical pharmacologist at the Lilly Laboratory for Clinical Research and held several positions during his time with the company, including Director of Clinical Research for Europe at Lilly Research Centre Limited, Erl Wood, UK, in 1985. Dr Zerbe became the Executive Director of the site, responsible for clinical investigation and regulatory affairs, in January 1989 and Vice President in June 1991, before moving to Parke-Davis Pharmaceutical Research in 1993. Dr Zerbe is a member of the Pharmaceutical Research and Manufacturers of America Medical Steering Committee, and the Commission on Drugs for Rare Diseases. He is also a Fellow of the American College of Physicians.

SECTION I

Introduction and Presentations

1 The application of toxicological investigations in the safe development of medicines

ROBERT ZERBE

Summary

1. One of the physician's primary roles in drug development is to provide a practical assessment of the risk and benefit from a clinical perspective. In doing this, the research physician must consider not only the benefit to the participating patient, but also the benefit derived for the population of patients with the disease under study.
2. In drug development, the physician is very dependent on the accuracy and validity of preclinical data. Preclinical studies should be as well conceived and executed as any clinical study, and results should be readily available to clinicians.
3. No single set of preclinical data requirements will apply to all situations. Many factors must be considered. These include the nature of the study participants, the expected human dose, the duration of treatment, trial design, the type and stage of disease to be treated, previous findings with the compound or related chemicals, and the magnitude of unmet medical need.
4. As clinicians, regulators, scientists and patients, we should resist the tendency to become more bureaucratic and conservative in drug development. Patients are waiting for innovative therapies, and highly risk averse standards which are rigidly applied to all situations will do more harm than good.

As part of this symposium, I would like to present a clinician's perspective on the non-clinical toxicology package, and to comment further on the wider role that toxicology studies play in the balance between regulations, litigation, responsibility to the patient and the need for rapid drug approval. To understand the research clinician's expectations of the preclinical data on which he bases clinical decisions, one must first appreciate the role that the clinician plays in the drug development process.

Clinicians as part of the drug development team

As part of the team, the clinician is expected to be an expert on the human disease which is to be studied. He is expected to know or have ready access to expert information which will allow timely decision-making and risk assessment. He is also expected to apply that knowledge to well conceived and innovative clinical research strategies which facilitate the advancement of science and speed the development of new drugs. The clinician will not be the sole contributor to clinical science on the team; in fact, many preclinical colleagues may be better informed about the pathogenesis and other aspects of the disease state. The critical knowledge which the clinician brings comes from the experience of clinical care which provides practical information frequently not found in textbooks and journals. Such practical information can be extremely important as one attempts to extrapolate preclinical data to a clinical setting.

The clinical research physician is the key link between the development team and the practising physician. In order to maintain that position, and use the association with the practising physician, whether he be an investigator or prescriber, to further the development of the drug, the research physician must carefully protect his credibility. He must be trusted to provide accurate and complete information to those physicians who are treating patients. The research physician is expected to represent the safety and well-being of patients first, regardless of the difficulty and controversy which may result. To the physician outside the company, the research physician is expected to blend his knowledge of pharmacology and drug development with medicine, so that the practising physician will be provided with well considered and unbiased guidance.

Because of his experience, the research physician is likely to be called upon as a good judge of risk and benefit to patients in clinical research. In clinical practice, the physician is routinely called upon to assess risks and benefits in considering therapeutic interventions for individual patients. The process in clinical research is the same, but the decision is complicated by uncertainty and complexity. The uncertainty stems from the experimental nature of the proposed treatments. In clinical practice, much is known about the therapeutic intervention and its likely effectiveness. In clinical research, it is not known whether the compound under study is either safe or effective. In clinical practice, the balance of risk and benefit rests within the patient. The patient both bears the risk and gains the benefit. In clinical research, the patient continues to bear the risk, but benefit may be generated for other patients as knowledge about the experimental compound is accumulated. The physician on the development team is well suited to deal with both the uncertainty and complexity of the decisions about human exposure that must be made.

The physician's expectations of preclinical data

Considering the importance of maintaining credibility and making valid judgements, the physician has high expectations of the preclinical data on which his statements and judgements are based. Since it is frequently hard to draw a clear and universally accepted line between some aspects of toxicology and other preclinical functions, I have taken the wider perspective and will consider the whole preclinical package as one.

Preclinical data, whether generated in toxicology or other preclinical departments, must be accurate and based on well conceived and well executed studies. Inaccurate data or poorly designed experiments can delay the development of the compound or, even worse, lead to misjudgements and potential harm to patients. Uninterpretable information does more harm than good, so as much thought must go into preclinical studies as clinical studies even though patients are not directly at risk.

The information presented to the physician must be comprehensive. Partial information can be very misleading, and the physician responsible for the clinical programme must be confident that all the preclinical findings have been shared. Often, the clinician does not have sufficient technical background to adequately assess the preclinical data, and depends on the preclinical scientist to provide an unbiased interpretation of the data. There is sometimes a very appropriate delay in the dissemination of preclinical data as they are reviewed and interpreted, but the research physician should be informed of even preliminary results if a critical clinical research decision is required before preclinical conclusions are reached.

Finally, the clinician expects some flexibility in the requirements for an adequate preclinical package. Considering the diverse situations in which the physician is asked to assess overall risk and benefit, it is unlikely that any single set of preclinical data requirements will fit all needs. In some situations, a smaller preclinical data set will not only be adequate but appropriate. Slowing development simply to satisfy a rigid requirement may be inappropriate when the drug under study has potential to save lives. On the other hand, even standard preclinical packages may not be adequate to minimise risks to patients under study. The preclinical scientists should work closely with the clinical scientists to craft an appropriately balanced preclinical programme to meet the clinicians' needs.

Preclinical data needs to support clinical testing

Many factors must be considered in the definition of an adequate preclinical package regardless of the stage of clinical development.

Study participants

The nature of the study participants may impact the type of preclinical data required. Healthy volunteers, or patients with mild or self-limited disease, have little to gain by the exposure to experimental compounds, and thus the development team must take special care to minimise risk through a comprehensive preclinical programme. Studies in children or fertile females will require special studies to assess potential risks to these populations. Though traditional approaches generally avoid exposure of such populations early in drug development, there is increasing pressure to be more inclusive and more complete in our evaluation of new compounds.

Expected human dose

There must be adequate preclinical data to cover the expected human dose. It is sometimes possible to predict the necessary dose or blood level which will be required for an appropriate clinical effect. This has been most common with anti-infectives for which efficacious blood levels can be predicted from preclinical work. As we develop more predictive surrogate markers in other disease states, our ability to predict adequate levels for clinical efficacy will improve. Our preclinical studies should cover such levels, if they can be predicted.

Duration of treatment

In many disease states, prolonged treatment may be necessary in order to adequately evaluate the efficacy of a drug. The preclinical data should be of sufficient duration to assess the adverse effects of such duration of exposure. Most investigators would advocate at least one preclinical day of exposure to cover one clinical day of exposure, but there is little scientific rationale for any specific standard.

Trial design

The type of trial or trial design may dictate certain additional preclinical studies in order to be safely executed. Adequate preclinical and clinical characterisation of the compound would be required before clinical experience trials could be initiated since such trials are likely to include a variety of patients with a wide spectrum of concomitant illnesses, of concomitant medications, and of disease severity. Combination therapy as part of a clinical study may require some evaluation of the acute toxicity of the combination, particularly if there are suggestions of such toxicity based on the pharmacology or metabolism of the combined drugs. Careful consideration of preclinical requirements for special studies will become more important as more innovative trial designs are developed in an effort to shorten drug development time lines.

Stage of disease

The stage of disease to be studied may be of importance in determining preclinical data needs. It is quite likely that the disease being treated may itself change the toxicity of the compound. One must raise the question of the need for more extensive toxicology and pharmacology in disease models. Considerable method development and validation would be required to confirm the relevance of such models to human disease, and in many such situations, no appropriate model would exist. On the other hand, it may be quite appropriate to require minimal toxicological data if a potentially life-saving medication is to be provided to a patient in the late stages of a terminal illness.

Previous findings

Special toxicology studies may be required if previous findings, with the study compound or another compound which is related pharmacologically or chemically, have indicated a special toxicological problem. In order to develop an adequate preclinical package, one must have a thorough understanding of other compounds in the therapeutic and chemical class, and it is particularly important to completely investigate and attempt to fully understand a toxicological problem when it is recognised.

Magnitude of unmet medical need

A final consideration in determining the size of the preclinical package is the magnitude of the unmet medical need. If the compound is likely to substantially improve the outcome in a severe disease for which there is no adequate therapy, some types of time-consuming toxicological testing should be temporarily waived. Such deviation from the rules will allow the medication to be made available to the patient who is in desperate need. This may come at some increased risk to the patient, but this added risk is far outweighed by potential benefit. Balancing risk and benefit will be discussed more fully later in this paper.

Preclinical data needs at various stages of clinical development

The purpose of this conference was to re-evaluate the specific toxicology studies required at various stages of clinical development. It is not the clinician's place to define the specific studies, but instead to outline the types of data which he needs to safely advance the development of the drug. In keeping with that theme, this section outlines the key decisions that the clinician must make and proposes the types of data needed to reach the best decision at each stage (Table 1.1). It is up to the toxicologists to determine how such information might be generated.

Initial single-dose studies in man

There are a number of responsibilities that the physician has when planning and executing initial dosing in man. Since this is the first exposure of humans, all data necessary to assess safety and minimise risk will obviously come from preclinical studies.

The clinician must first select a safe starting dose. This is generally determined by taking some conservative fraction of the dose which had no detectable effect in animals. This no-effect dose should generally be determined in more than one species since any single species may show substantially different pharmacological or metabolic characteristics of the drug.

The clinician should have sufficient information from a preclinical data package to anticipate the type of toxicity which he might encounter as the dose in humans is escalated. Knowing what toxicities to anticipate enables the physician to monitor carefully for types of toxicities and respond early in order to avoid any severe toxicity in man. This also allows the clinician to plan a strategy for reversal of the toxicities should they occur. This calls for multiple species characterisation of acute toxicity in animals and, when possible, some preclinical evaluation of methods to reverse the toxic effects.

It is useful for the clinician to have a reasonable idea of the anticipated dose or blood level which will produce the desired pharmacological effect. If this can be done with a reasonable degree of certainty, the clinician may be able to stop dose escalation before encountering clinical toxicity; this is something which should always be avoided if possible. In order to adequately predict the

Table 1.1 Preclinical data requirements at each stage of clinical development

Clinical Stage	*Preclinical Data*
Initial single-dose study	No effect dose in >1 species Multiple species characterisation of acute and repeated dose toxicity Preclinical evaluation of methods to reverse toxic effects Pharmacological profile Genotoxicity Metabolic and kinetic characterisation in >1 species Special studies, depending on patient population
Multiple-dose safety studies	Multiple-dose toxicity in >1 species of a minimum duration = clinical exposure Characterisation of toxicity of parent and metabolites Toxicity of related compounds
Long-term efficacy and safety trials (beyond Phase I)	Multiple-dose toxicity in >1 species of a minimum duration = clinical exposure Special studies of synthesised metabolite, if no test species produces the human metabolite In some cases, pharmacodynamic interaction studies Special studies, depending on patient population

pharmacological dose in man, a good pharmacological profile must be developed as part of the preclinical data package.

The clinician must have sufficient data to feel confident that even short-term exposure will not lead to latent toxicities in man. Thus, even single doses in man should be covered by repeat dosing in more than one animal species. It is also appropriate to evaluate the potential for genotoxicity prior to single-dose studies. The probability of a single dose producing latent toxicities seems quite low, but considering most initial dosing is done in normal volunteers, minimisation of the potential risk is required to balance the negligible benefit in such subjects.

The preclinical package should allow the physician to make a reasonable prediction of the metabolism and kinetics of the compound. Adequate characterisation of the kinetics and metabolism early in clinical studies is becoming increasingly important. Being able to reasonably predict the kinetics and metabolism in man enables optimisation of the trial design and sampling intervals. Thus, ever more detailed metabolic and kinetic characterisation in more than one preclinical species will assist in clinical trial design.

If special populations, such as fertile women, are to be used in initial dosing, special toxicity studies will be required. These studies might include fertility studies and studies of embryotoxicity. Other populations such as children or patients with multiple concomitant medications may also require special preclinical studies.

Multiple-dose safety studies

The physician, having been assured of reasonable safety in single-dose studies, moves to multiple-dose safety evaluations. One of the major features of such trials which must be determined is the dose and dosing interval. This is largely based on the results of the single-dose study and the intended clinical dose if that has been determined. The preclinical studies necessary for the physician to be confident in the dose and duration chosen are multiple-dose toxicity studies in more than one animal species. Having obtained an initial indication about the metabolism in man, it is possible to choose an appropriate animal model in which exposure to both the parent and metabolites has been evaluated from a toxicological perspective. In the future, one might actually consider fewer species in toxicity studies if those species can be shown to mimic man with respect to metabolism and kinetics.

The physician should have enough information to anticipate potential toxicities after multiple dosing. The duration of toxicological studies to support multiple-dose safety evaluation in man varies from country to country. The duration should be sufficient to detect adverse effects of drug accumulation and latent toxicity, and a minimum of one day per day of clinical exposure would be essential. In order to properly anticipate clinical toxicities, the physician should not only know the preclinical data generated for the compound under study, but also be knowledgeable about the toxicities of related compounds. In this regard, special preclinical studies of related compounds can be very helpful to the clinician when trying to extrapolate observed toxicities from the laboratory to the clinic.

Long-term efficacy and safety trials (beyond Phase I)

Since most studies in Phase I are done in normal volunteers, progression to Phase II generally represents the first exposure to patients, and thus additional preclinical data may be required. In addition, the duration of exposure is usually much longer to allow adequate evaluation of both safety and efficacy.

The choice of the dose or doses in these trials is generally determined by previous clinical experience with the drug in man. Toxicology dosing should have produced sufficiently high blood levels of the drug and the human metabolites in order to provide a reasonable safety margin. If no species produces the human metabolites, special toxicology studies of the synthesised metabolite may be necessary.

The duration of such studies is dictated by the time of exposure required to properly assess efficacy and by regulatory requirements for sufficient patient exposure to assess safety. A consensus on the duration of clinical exposure required to conclude that a compound is reasonably safe has emerged from the Second International Conference on Harmonisation (ICH2) but has not been uniformly implemented. Generally, chronic medications require a minimum of a few hundred patients for at least one year. In general, physicians would probably feel most comfortable with a minimum of one day of toxicology exposure for each day of clinical exposure, but this obviously becomes less important as the duration of patient treatment increases. The clinical relevance of prolonged exposure of very high doses of the compound to animals for prolonged periods is unknown.

Moving into clinical studies in patients also introduces the problem of concomitant medications and illnesses. At this stage of development, the clinical and preclinical data should have provided sufficient information on the pathways of metabolism that major drug interactions could be predicted. A variety of preclinical *in vitro* approaches hold promise in this area. In some situations preclinical pharmacodynamic interaction studies would be desirable prior to the initiation of the studies.

Concomitant illnesses present a more significant problem. It is not common for disease/drug interactions to be evaluated in the preclinical laboratory since preclinical models are frequently not relevant to the clinical situation. This may be an important area for toxicology development in the future.

As mentioned above, populations of women, children and elderly patients may require special data, some of which would be generated in the preclinical laboratory.

A number of unanswered questions arise out of this discussion as well. Considering the advancement in analytical methods, are we fully utilising metabolic data to decrease animal exposure by intensively studying a smaller number of more relevant species? Are long-term toxicology data actually contributing much to our knowledge, or is there a better way to obtain comparable data? Could clinical development be more rational and rapid by developing and utilising more surrogate markers of efficacy in the preclinical and clinical studies? Is there value in attempting to better understand drug-disease interactions in the preclinical setting? Could toxicology requirements be altered if we were to move more exclusively to patients who have the potential to benefit from trial participation, rather than normal volunteers who have little to gain?

Summary of the clinician's needs from the preclinical laboratory

In this paper, only a broad description of the types of data required to assist the physician in clinical development have been presented, but some general observations are worth summarising. First, pre-clinical data must be accurate and comprehensive. Second, toxicology data, even with its understandable limitations, is important to the clinician, particularly early in development. Last, in defining toxicology data needs, we should consider the questions that need to be answered, not the boxes that need to be checked.

Balancing risk and benefit

The physician is the individual on the development team who is most likely to be called upon to assess the balance of risk and benefit of any development strategy involving patients. This responsibility stems not only from his knowledge of patient care, but also from his experience in clinical practice in which he routinely assesses risk and benefit, and chooses a course of action.

The assessment of risk and benefit in clinical research is, however, more complicated than that in clinical practice. In the latter, the patient nearly always shares both the risk and benefit of any therapy. Thus, the risk to the patient, whether it is high or low, must be outweighed by the benefit provided to that patient. In clinical research, the patient participating in the programme will bear the risk, and in most cases the patient will derive a benefit which outweighs any risk which he bears. In some cases, however, the benefit to the patient may be modest, and the primary beneficiaries are the population of patients who are inadequately treated by current therapies. In clinical research, the total benefit, including that generated for individuals not participating directly in the trial must be considered. Undue risk to the individual patient, obviously, cannot be tolerated regardless of the benefit to the population as a whole.

There are many situations in which considerable potential benefit may come to a patient as the result of participation in a trial. These situations would include terminal, life threatening or severely disabling diseases. If such therapies are delayed in order to decrease risk (i.e. while additional toxicological data are collected) less benefit is generated for both the study patient and the afflicted population which would benefit from earlier availability. Therefore, compounds with great potential for meeting an unmet medical need should move forward quickly in development even if there is a modest increase in overall risk. On the other hand, compounds which do little to improve medical care, should be shown to have very low risk. It is therefore reasonable to propose that no single standard of toxicology requirements will meet the needs in all situations.

Determining where we are, as a regulated industry, on the risk/benefit balance would probably be the result of a long and heated debate, if it could be done at all. There are some examples of accelerated development of treatments for high profile diseases such as AIDS. Development of therapies for less politicised but equally disastrous diseases such as cancer have been painfully slow. On balance, it is probably fair to say that with the exception of a few prominent diseases, drug development has been slowed by a progressively more conservative approach. The guidelines become more demanding following each publicised adverse finding with a drug. Functionally, the guidelines become rules for adequate investigation, and all companies slavishly follow them for fear of litigation or later embarrassment. The unfortunate outcome of this replacement of science with bureaucracy is that rational drug development is not allowed to set the right balance between risk and benefit.

The evolution toward less rational, less consistent and less innovative regulatory positions is not confined to drug regulation, nor is it solely the fault of the regulators. Stephen Breyer in his book *Breaking the Vicious Circle*, describes a similar process for all regulatory agencies dealing with risk.

The vicious circle starts with a public which is very poor at understanding and balancing risk. There are numerous explanations for this. People use heuristic devices to oversimplify very complex situations. People react most to prominent situations such as those carried in the mass media. People are strongly influenced by personal situations such as sick patients. People are becoming progressively more distrustful of experts. People tend to make up their minds quickly, and are reluctant to change them. In addition to the psychological characteristics, people lack the skills in mathematics and probability to adequately understand the complexity of health risk and benefit.

The legislators over-react to adverse situations. Whether they do so with good intentions or for political gain, they step in with legislation which attempts to solve complex problems with detailed rules, the adverse impact of which they do not appreciate.

The regulators are left with little choice but to comply with the law, and when thrust into a process filled with high uncertainty, they move to a very conservative posture to avoid potential for error. Companies are equally risk averse where a sensational press, hostile special interest groups and trial lawyers thrive. The unfortunate outcome of all this is that the patients that need new therapies most are denied them because we live in a society which has grown to avoid risk above all else.

The benefits of bringing a more rational balance between risk and benefit into the development of new drugs would extend beyond more rapid availability. It would also allow more effective utilisation of drug development resources so that more treatments could be made available. It would also allow the more rapid evolution of medical knowledge, enabling increased probability of medical breakthroughs and better preparation for emerging medical problems.

This series of papers is an excellent opportunity to make a small contribution to bringing risk and benefit back to a more scientific footing. Along those lines, as recommendations for toxicology guidelines are considered, we should advocate flexibility in guidelines which allow the toxicology programme to be tailored to the needs of the situation.

References

Breyer S (1993). *Breaking the Vicious Circle. Toward Effective Risk Regulation.* Harvard University Press, Cambridge, Mass.

2 Review of international recommendations on animal toxicity studies and their relation to clinical exposure

DAVID SCALES and TOSHIMI USUI

Summary

1. The current guidelines on animal repeated dose toxicity, oncogenicity, genetic toxicity, reproductive toxicity and antigenicity studies related to clinical exposure are reviewed for Japan, the European Union and the USA.

2. Major differences are seen between the three regions with respect to repeated dose studies, with shorter duration animal toxicity studies being required to support clinical studies in the USA compared with the rest of the world. There are some differences in oncogenicity requirements and the genotoxicity package for marketing authorisation is currently being discussed within the ICH Expert Working Group. The reproductive toxicology package differs between the three regions although Segment I male fertility will probably now not be required prior to Phase I clinical studies with male subjects.

3. Full toxicology reports are required for marketing applications in Japan, the USA and the EU. The USA also requires full reports for an IND, whereas in Japan and in most EU States, summaries are usually adequate.

4. The authors conclude that for a multinational company, it may currently be advantageous to conduct initial clinical studies in Europe, extend the clinical programme by conducting clinical studies in the USA and then apply for first marketing authorisation in Europe and the USA.

This paper represents a synthesis of custom and practice, current guidelines as well as recommendations made following the First International Conference on Harmonisation (ICH1) in 1991 and ICH2 in 1993.

Single-dose toxicity

Single-dose studies, in two rodent species, by the clinical route plus one other route (usually intravenous if the clinical is not the intravenous route) are recommended before human studies.

Repeat-dose toxicity

In support of clinical trials

Table 2.1 summarises current regulatory practice. The duration of toxicity studies refer to a rodent plus a non-rodent, usually rat and

Table 2.1 Repeated dose toxicity requirements in support of clinical studies

	Minimum toxicology requirement		
Proposed duration of clinical study	*Japan*[*1]	*EU*[2]	*USA*[3]
1 day		2 weeks	For Phase I & II
3 days			
7 days	1 month	1 month	Clinical = Toxicology Duration
30 days	3 months	3 months	
>30 days	6 months	6 months	For Phase III
≥3 months			
>6 months			Clinical = ⅓ Toxicology Duration

*In the absence of specific guidance on toxicology requirements in support of clinical trials in Japan,[4] the Japanese marketing requirements[1] are utilised according to customary practice.
[1]MHW: Guidelines for Toxicity Studies of Drugs, 1989.
[2]CPMP: Recommendations for the Development of Non-Clinical Testing Strategies, Draft 7, July 1990.
[3]PMA: Guidelines for the Assessment of Drug and Medical Device Safety in Animals, February 1977. Custom & Practice.
[4]MHW: General Guideline for Clinical Evaluation of New Drugs Draft 4, August 1988.

dog. In the USA the phase of the clinical study is taken into account, Phase I and Phase II study duration can equal the duration of the toxicology studies. For Phase III the clinical study duration can extend to 1/3 of the toxicology duration. Thus 3-month toxicity studies support a 1-month clinical study. In the USA, clinical studies of over three months should be supported by 6-month studies. A 12-month dog study is not usually required until a New Drug Application (NDA).

In support of marketing applications

Repeat-dose studies for marketing applications are summarised in Table 2.2. As in Table 2.1, the toxicology durations refer to studies on a rodent and non-rodent. Twelve-month studies in dogs, following the recommendations of ICH1, are now only required by the Food and Drug Administration (FDA) in cases where the medicine will be given for over three months. The European Union (EU) still does not require 12-month studies, and the Ministry of Health and Welfare (MHW) has amended its guidelines to delete the requirement for such studies. It should be noted that the minimum duration for a toxicity study in Japan is one month, compared to two weeks for the EU and the USA.

Table 2.2 Repeated dose toxicity requirements in support of marketing

	Minimum toxicology requirement		
Proposed clinical duration	*Japan*[1]	*EU*[2]	*USA*[3]
1 day		2 weeks	2 weeks
3 days			
7 days	1 month	1 month	
30 days	3 months	3 months	13 weeks
>30 days	6 months	6 months	
3 months			26 weeks
>3 months			52 weeks or longer
>6 months			

[1]MHW: Guidelines for Toxicity Studies of Drugs, 1989.
[2]CPMP: Repeated Dose Toxicity, October 1983.
[3]PMA: Guidelines for the Assessment of Drug and Medical Device Safety in Animals, February 1977.

Oncogenicity studies

Table 2.3 summarises current regulatory practice with regard to oncogenicity testing. EU member states have differing recommendations concerning clinical trials. It is interesting to note that in Norway (Nordic Council on Medicines, 1983), oncogenicity studies should be completed prior to exceeding six months clinical duration. However, more recently, the Swedish authorities have amended this requirement and will not normally request carcinogenicity data when assessing trials of shorter duration than one year (Medical Products Agency, 1992). In the UK, such studies are required, in the MAL 4 guidelines, prior to exceeding 12 months (Department of Health and Social Security, 1984). The Medicines Control Agency (MCA), however, does not enforce this requirement and the clinical trial guidelines in the UK are currently under review. In Ireland,

Table 2.3 Oncogenicity

	Marketing requirements	*Clinical trial requirements*
USA	Recommended for most drugs[1] exceptions in practice being drugs intended for short-term use only (i.e. for under 3 months)	Only when there is cause for concern[1]
Japan	When there is cause for concern or when long-term clinical use is expected[2] (i.e. over 6 months)	Recommended (but not usually done) prior to Phase III, according to market requirements criteria[3]
EU	When there is cause for concern or when long-term clinical use is expected[4] (i.e. over 6 months)	Recommended as per marketing requirements[5] but not usually done prior to long-term clinical studies unless suspicions arise

[1]PMA: Guidelines for the Assessment of Drug and Medical Device Safety in Animals, February 1977.
[2]MHW: Guidelines for Toxicity Studies of Drugs, 1989.
[3]MHW: General Guidelines for Clinical Evaluation of New Drugs (Draft), 4 August 1988.
[4]CPMP: Carcinogenic Potential, October 1983.
[5]CPMP: Recommendations for the Development of Non-Clinical Testing Strategies, Draft No. 7, 5 July 1990.

oncogenicity studies should be "well under way" before exceeding six months clinical exposure (National Drugs Advisory Board, 1991).

The top dose for oncogenicity studies for the FDA does not now have to be the maximum tolerated dose, but can have an upper limit at a minimum of 25 times the human AUC (area under the curve of plasma concentration vs time curve) (FDA, 1994).

Genetic toxicity

The various recommendations in current guidelines and draft guidelines on genetic toxicology are summarised in Table 2.4. The ICH Expert Working Group is actively debating what studies are required before human exposure. An agreed core test battery is anticipated by ICH3. Current custom and practice in most areas is to perform a bacterial test such as an Ames test for gene mutation and a test for chromosome damage prior to human exposure. Some companies are completing all genotoxicity studies before exceeding one month's clinical exposure. The inclusion of *in vitro* gene mutation tests, e.g. the mouse lymphoma assay, is being considered by the ICH Group.

Table 2.4 Genetic toxicity

	Marketing requirements	*Clinical trial requirements*
Japan	3 test package[1]	'Fundamental part' of test package prior to Phase I[2]
USA	No specific recommendations	No specific recommendations
EU	3 or 4 test package[3] (usually 4 unless the drug is an antimicrobial)	3 or 4 test package recommended[4] but only Ames (and often micronucleus) test routinely done before human exposure

[1]MHW: Guidelines for Toxicity Studies of Drugs, 1989.
[2]MHW: General Guidelines for Clinical Evaluation of New Drugs (Draft), 4 August 1988.
[3]CPMP: Testing of Medicinal Products for their Mutagenic Potential, February 1987.
[4]CPMP: Recommendations for the Development of Non-Clinical Testing Strategies, Draft No. 7, 5 July 1990.

Reproductive toxicity

Marketing requirements

A Step 4 ICH document entitled "Detection of Toxicity to Reproduction for Medicinal Products", detailing the various test options required for the marketing of a drug was issued on 24th June 1993. The marketing requirements in Japan, the USA and the EU are therefore harmonised.

Table 2.5 Reproductive toxicity

	Clinical trial requirements	
	Male subjects	*Female subjects*
EU	No specific recommendations	Only Segment II in rodent and non-rodent done routinely by this stage
Japan	*Male portion of Segment I prior to Phase I[1]	All 3 segments plus prior evidence of clinical safety and efficacy in males[1]; in practice, Segment III not done routinely by this stage USA
USA	No specific recommendations	Segment II in rodent and non-rodent plus female portion of Segment I[2,3], prior evidence of clinical safety and efficacy in males (all 3 segments before large-scale trials)[3]

[1]MHW: General Guidelines for Clinical Evaluation of New Drugs (Draft), 4 August 1988
[2]PMA: Guidelines for the Assessment of Drug and Medical Device Safety in Animals, February 1977.
[3]FDA: General Considerations for the Clinical Evaluation of Drugs, September 1977.

*With regard to male fertility studies in Japan, this was discussed in March 1994 at an ICH meeting in Tokyo. The results of a joint investigation between the Japan Pharmaceutical Manufacturers Association (JPMA) and the Japanese Ministry of Health and Welfare (MHW) were presented, including detailed histopathological findings regarding testicular changes and the spermatogenesis associated with several compounds. Professor Omori reported that the histopathological techniques are very sensitive methods for detecting changes in the testis, which, in turn, probably reflect almost all changes in reproductive organs. Therefore, Segment I studies should not be required prior to a Phase I clinical trial in Japan. This has not yet been officially announced. Meanwhile, some Japanese companies are still doing Segment I studies before clinical trials while others are not.

Clinical trial requirements

The ICH Step 4 document does not address the types of study required for clinical trials. The current regulatory practice in this area is given in Table 2.5. In the USA, there is a move to include females at an earlier stage in the development programme. Segment I, II and III studies routinely use the rat, whereas the Segment II non-rodent is usually the rabbit.

Table 2.6 Recommendations for additional toxicological studies

	Juvenile toxicology prior to paediatric trials	*Antigenicity testing*	*Studies on human metabolites*
Japan	Recommended[1]	Package of investigations[2] recommended prior to human trials, particularly for external or parenteral drugs[3] in addition to sensitisation testing	Animal toxicology on main human metabolites recommended[2]
USA	Recommended[4]	Sensitisation testing recommended for dermally applied drugs5	No specific recommendations
EU	Suggested[6], but not routinely done	Sensitisation testing recommended for dermally applied drugs[7]	Investigate suspicious metabolites in animals or man8

[1]MHW: Guideline for Development of Paediatric Drugs, 1981.
[2]Yakugo Jiho: Drug Approval and Licensing Procedures in Japan.
[3]MHW: General Guideline for Clinical Evaluation of New Drugs (draft), 4 August 1988.
[4]FDA: General Considerations for the Clinical Evaluation of Drugs in Infants and Children, Sept. 1977.
[5]PMA: Guidelines for the Assessment of Drug and Medical Device Safety in Animals, Feb. 1977.
[6]CPMP: Clinical Investigation of Medicinal Products in Children, September 1988.
[7]CPMP: Non-Clinical Local Tolerance Testing of Medicinal Products, 12 December 1990.
[8]CPMP: Pharmacokinetic Studies in Man, February 1987.

Additional studies

Additional studies required for medicinal products are outlined in Table 2.6.

To date, the MHW has required antigenicity tests for all newly developed drugs. However, in March 1994 at the ICH Expert Working Group meeting in Tokyo, the JPMA had a meeting with the MHW concerning the international harmonisation of antigenicity studies. At that meeting the responsible officers of the MHW mentioned that they would revise the present guidelines for both toxicity testing and marketing applications concerning antigenicity studies so that these studies would become optional. Their conduct would then be dependent on the individual company's decision, on a case by case basis.

Single-dose studies on the main human metabolites are still recommended for Japanese applications.

Report requirements

Full toxicology reports are required for marketing applications in Japan, the USA and the EU. The USA also requires full reports for an IND, whereas in Japan, and in most EU member states, summaries are usually adequate.

It is our understanding that the publication of preclinical data in Japan in Japanese, specifically single- and repeat-dose as well as reproductive and developmental toxicity, has been reviewed by the MHW. The only requirement now is to publish key studies actually carried out in Japan.

Effect upon development programme

Currently it is more expeditious to start single-dose studies in males in the EU because:

1. There are no recommendations for male reproductive toxicity testing;
2. Only summaries of reports are required, unlike in the USA; and
3. 14 days toxicity testing is recommended compared to one month in Japan.

Inclusion of women in the clinical programme is also more expeditious in the EU because there are no recommendations for female fertility testing, unlike in the USA and Japan.

However, when the duration of trials is extended it is more expeditious to conduct them in the USA because Phase I and Phase II clinical testing only requires toxicology studies equal to the duration of clinical use, whereas six months is recommended in the EU and Japan for trials of over four weeks' duration.

Conclusion

In summary, the suggestion is that for a multinational pharmaceutical company it may be advantageous to conduct initial clinical studies in Europe, extend the clinical programme by conducting clinical studies in the USA and then apply for first marketing authorisation in Europe and the USA.

References

Department of Health and Social Security (DHSS) (1984). Medicines Act 1968. Guidance Notes on Applications for Clinical Trials Certificates and Clinical Trials Exemptions. HMSO.

Food and Drug Administration (FDA) (1994). *Federal Register*, March 1, 1994, Docket No 94D-0017.

Medical Products Agency (1992). Regarding requirements for carcinogenicity data in support of clinical trials of long term duration. Högaktuellt. Läkemedelsverket – Nyhetsblad i registreringsfrägor No 8, March 1992.

National Drugs Advisory Board (1991). Guidelines for Application for Clinical Trial Investigations of Medicinal Products for Human Use.

Nordic Council on Medicines (1983). Clinical trials of drugs. NLN-publication No. 11. Ed June 1983

3 International survey on the timing of toxicity studies in relation to clinical trials

CHRISTOPHER PARKINSON

Summary

1. A questionnaire-based survey of pharmaceutical companies is being conducted to: (i) ascertain companies' current approaches and views on an ideal approach to the timing of toxicity studies in relation to clinical investigation; (ii) highlight current problems resulting from the differences in national guidelines in this area; (iii) provide an overview of the international situation, contributing to discussions aimed towards rationalising the timing of toxicity studies.
2. The results of preliminary analyses on the data provided by 30 companies show that a wide range of toxicology strategies are currently used by companies in their development of new medicines.
3. There is also a wide range of proposed ideal approaches to the topic which suggests that different toxicology strategies are adopted due to differences in scientific and strategic thinking as well as for regulatory reasons.
4. Two areas of the timing of toxicity testing that stand out as having diverse scientific approaches are the reproductive studies carried out before including women in clinical trials and the need for carcinogenicity tests to support Phase III.
5. This survey is providing data important for establishing a baseline from which to develop an industry consensus, leading to future international harmonisation on the timing of toxicity studies in relation to clinical trials.

Introduction

The recommendations for the extent of non-clinical testing to support the various stages of clinical development frequently differ between the regions of Europe, Japan and the USA (Scales and Mahoney, 1991). For those companies choosing to implement a multinational clinical testing programme, this raises the important issue of whether there is any scientific justification for these differences in guidelines. If not, what would be the minimum acceptable, scientifically justifiable set of toxicity studies needed to progress into each phase of clinical development? This question is being discussed in 1994 by the Committee for Proprietary Medicinal Products (CPMP) Safety Working Party to bring about some harmonisation within Europe and it is also a topic for the Third International Conference on Harmonisation (ICH3). Resolution of these differences in regulations will allow companies to optimise their toxicity testing strategy to suit the developmental needs for individual compounds.

There could be significant advantages in resolving this harmonisation issue if an international pharmaceutical industry consensus was available at an early stage. As yet, however, complete agreement amongst the international pharmaceutical industry on a common approach to the timing of toxicity studies has not been reached. To aid discussions towards this industry consensus, it is important to have data on the current strategies being used by companies and to obtain a broad representation of views on what is considered to be an ideal approach. A survey has therefore been conducted to address these needs.

Survey methodology and response

The objective of the survey was to collect data on the whole spectrum of toxicity testing and when, in relation to clinical development, these studies are carried out by international pharmaceutical companies. A questionnaire was devised which allowed respondents to indicate their company's current practice regarding the toxicity studies initiated and completed, or in the case of repeated dose studies, the duration of the toxicity test completed, at various defined steps in clinical development. Information on a number of factors affecting the choice and implementation of a strategy was

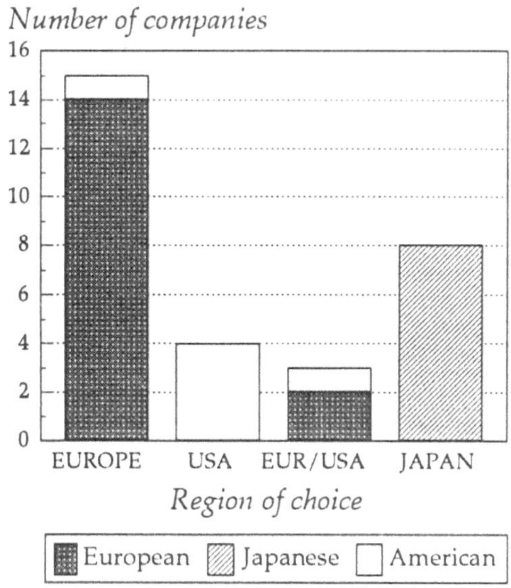

Figure 3.1 Choice of location for initial Phase I studies by European, Japanese and American companies

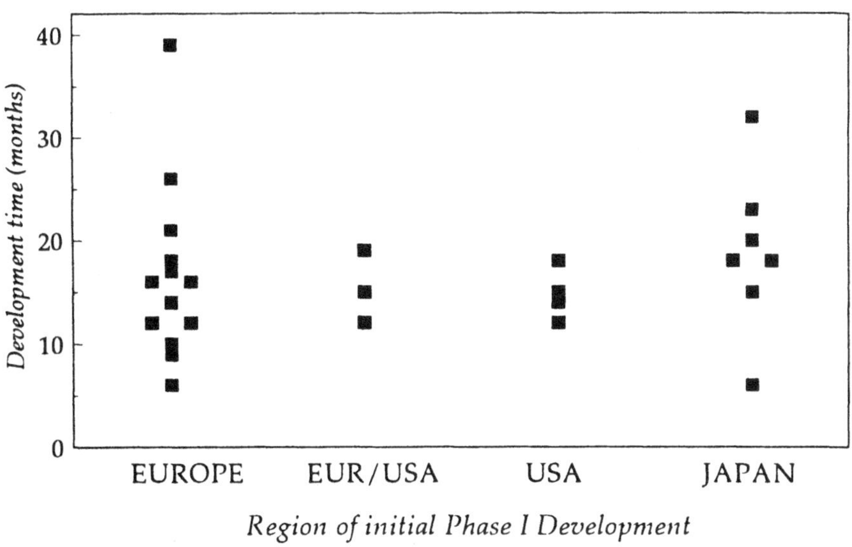

Figure 3.2 Time taken from identification of a candidate drug for development to the first administration to man for clinical development in Japan, the USA, Europe or simultaneously in Europe and the USA (each symbol represents the average for one company)

also requested including whether the compound was for short- or long-term use, the choice of location of development and other internal or external factors such as rate-limiting steps in the development process. Respondents were also asked to indicate their suggested ideal approach to a toxicity testing strategy, that is, what they would like to do in an unregulated situation. The questionnaire was sent to 67 pharmaceutical companies and their subsidiaries, representing 54 company groups in Europe, Japan and the United States.

A preliminary analysis was conducted on data from 30 companies (16 from Europe, 8 from Japan and 6 from the USA) on the development of compounds for long-term use. Three initial areas of investigation were chosen for the analysis:

- Toxicity studies conducted before the first administration to humans;
- The duration of repeated dose toxicity studies conducted to support all phases of clinical development;
- The timing of reproductive toxicity testing.

Results

Initiating Phase I studies

Most companies use their home region for initiating Phase I studies (Figure 3.1) for several reasons, including the convenience of being situated in the same local region, the fact that they have developed their facilities in this area and for marketing or regulatory reasons. Three companies (two European and one American) initiate Phase I studies simultaneously in Europe and the USA. One American company initiates Phase I in Europe because of the lack of a requirement for an investigational new drug (IND) filing in Europe. It has been suggested that compounds can be taken into man more quickly in Europe than in other regions because of this lack of regulation (Scales and Mahoney, 1991). Data collected to date, however, showed a broad range of times taken from the identification of a candidate drug for development to the first administration to humans with little overall differences between regions (Figure 3.2).

Toxicity testing to support the first administration to man

Acute toxicity testing

All companies conduct acute toxicity studies before a compound is used in man for the first time and more than half indicated that acute studies or high dose safety pharmacology would be included in their ideal toxicity testing strategy.

Genetic toxicology

Companies currently conduct a range of different genetic toxicology packages before initiating Phase I studies (Figure 3.3A). Only three companies responding complete an Ames or bacterial mutation test on its own. Generally, most of the companies do an Ames test in conjunction with one or more other tests such as an *in vitro* or *in vivo*

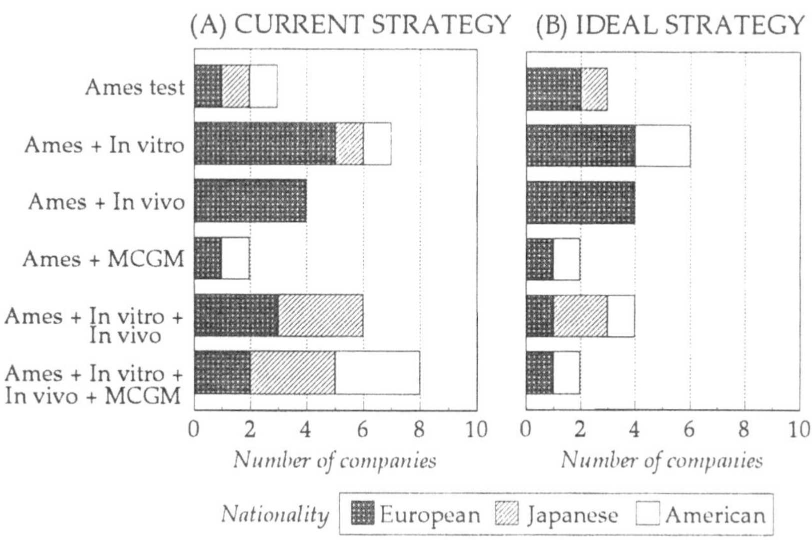

Key:
In vitro = in vitro cytogenetics
In vivo = in vivo cytogenetics (e.g. micronucleus)
MCGM = mammalian cell gene mutation (e.g. mouse lymphoma test)

Figure 3.3 Genotoxicity studies conducted as part of current (A) or ideal (B) toxicity testing strategy to support the first administration of a new medicine to humans

cytogenicity test or the mammalian cell gene mutation assay. Eight of the 30 responding companies, mainly Japanese or American, complete all four components of the genetic toxicology package at this stage. However, fewer companies considered that conducting all four tests was the ideal approach, with the majority preferring some combination of an Ames (bacterial mutation) test plus one or two cytogenicity tests as the ideal preclinical genetic toxicology package (Figure 3.3B).

Repeated dose and reproductive toxicity studies

In addition to genotoxicity testing and acute toxicity studies, all companies currently carry out some repeated dose toxicology, ranging from 14- to 90-day studies, before the first administration of a new medicine to man (Figure 3.4A). In general, 14-day repeated dose studies are conducted mainly by American companies whereas 1-month studies tend to be carried out by European and Japanese companies. Two Japanese companies carry out 90-day studies. Some companies, mostly Japanese but including four European, also complete certain reproductive toxicity studies before going into Phase I. In the case of Japanese companies, this is usually a rodent fertility study and some may even include with this an embryo/foetal toxicity study.

A different picture exists for the ideal strategy (Figure 3.4B). The main differences are that a number of the European companies would ideally complete a 14-day rather than a 1-month repeated dose study and those European companies currently conducting reproductive toxicology at this stage would not to do so in an ideal situation.

Animal toxicity studies to support repeated dosing in humans

Companies have a wide range of approaches with respect to repeated dose toxicity testing to support the various stages of clinical development (Table 3.1). The duration of toxicity studies currently completed by companies prior to initiating Phase III ranges from three months (for one Japanese company) up to the long-term tests for carcinogenicity (8 companies; 5 European, 1 American and 2 Japanese).

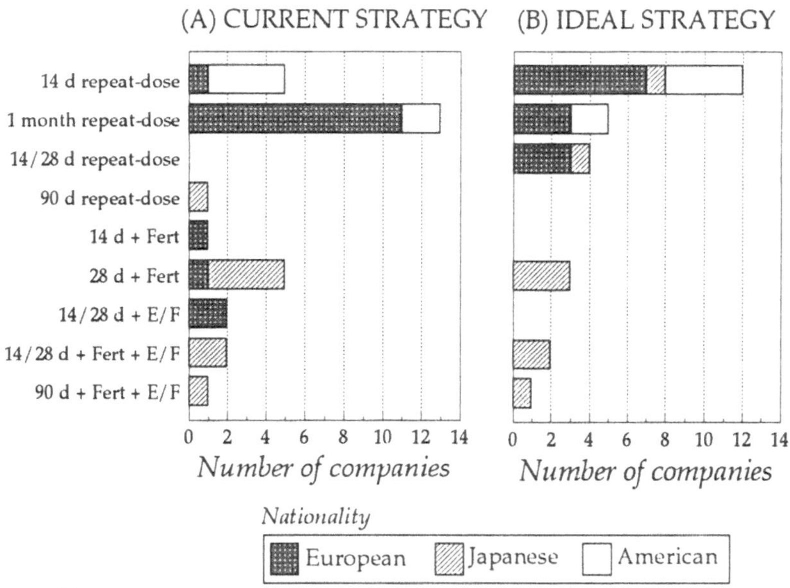

Key:
E/F = Embryo/foetal developmental toxicity study
Fert = Fertility study
d = day

Figure 3.4 Repeated dose and reproductive toxicity studies conducted as part of current (A) or ideal (B) toxicity testing strategy to support the initial investigation of a new medicine in humans

Table 3.1 Single- and repeated dose toxicity studies currently completed by companies to support various stages of clinical development

	No of companies completing animal toxicity studies of a maximum duration of:						
Clinical duration	14 days	1 mo	3 mo	6 mo	6/12 mo*	12 mo	24 mo**
Single dose	8	20	2	–	–	–	–
Up to 1 week	2	22	6	–	–	–	–
Up to 1 month	–	2	16	12	–	–	–
Up to 6 months	–	–	2	17	8	3	–
Phase III	–	–	1	9	8	4	8

* 6-month study in rodents and 12-month study in non-rodents
** carcinogenicity study

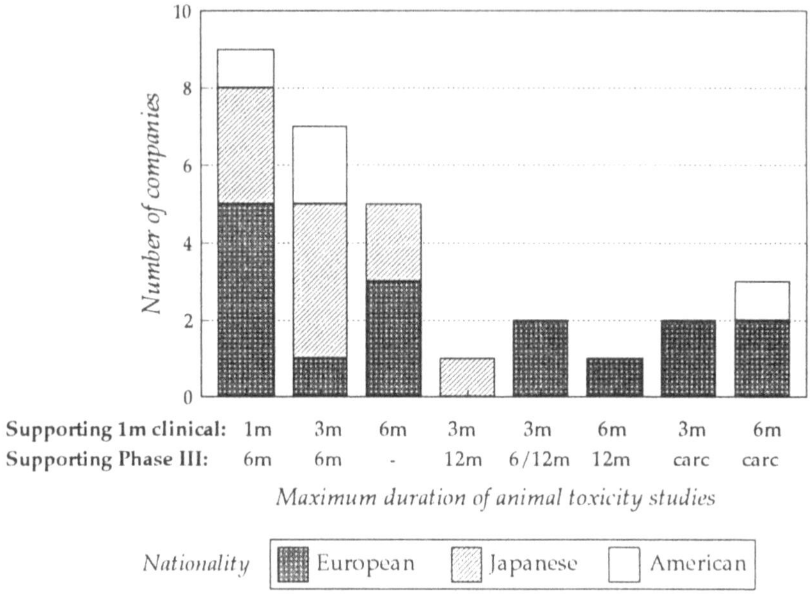

6/12 denotes 6-month study in rodents and 12-month study in non-rodents.
carc = 2-year study for carcinogenicity; m = months

Figure 3.5 Ideal repeated dose toxicity testing strategies suggested by companies to support clinical use of up to one month and subsequent initiation of Phase III

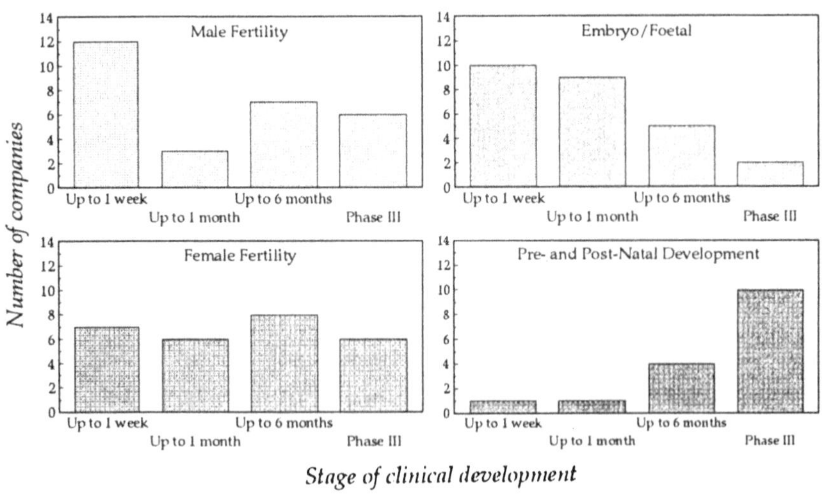

Figure 3.6 Stages in clinical development prior to which companies currently complete the four aspects of reproductive and developmental toxicity testing

Figure 3.5 shows the maximum duration of repeated dose toxicity studies suggested by companies as an ideal approach to supporting 1-month and Phase III clinical trials. The most favoured approach (16 companies) was to conduct 1- or 3-month repeated dose toxicology to support clinical trials up to one month followed by 6-month toxicity studies to support the initiation of Phase III clinical trials. For five companies, the ideal strategy was to complete 6-month studies in support of 1-month clinical trials which would then allow progression into Phase III without any further repeated dose toxicology being done. Five other companies (4 European and 1 American) would ideally complete at least one carcinogenicity study before initiating Phase III clinical trials. The amount of repeated dose toxicology these companies would ideally carry out to support 1-month clinical trials varied between three and six months.

The timing of reproductive toxicity testing

There were large differences seen between companies regarding the stage of development at which the four studies that constitute the reproductive toxicity testing package (male fertility, female fertility, embryo/foetal toxicity and pre- and post-natal development) were completed (Figure 3.6). Apart from the eight Japanese companies who conduct male fertility studies prior to one week administration in the clinic, the remaining companies as a whole showed no particular preference for any stage of clinical development at which they conduct fertility studies. The embryo/foetal toxicity study is conducted at an early stage of development by more companies and the pre- and post-natal development study is performed later; nearly 50% of the companies having not completed this prior to initiation of Phase III trials.

The reproductive toxicity package completed by companies prior to including females in clinical trials for the first time was also characterised by a number of different approaches in current strategies (Figure 3.7A). Eleven companies (8 European and 3 American) consider an embryo/foetal developmental toxicity study to be sufficient at this stage. However, 12 companies, including all of the Japanese, carry out more than this. One Japanese company completes a carcinogenicity study prior to inclusion of women in clinical trials, in addition to the whole of the reproductive testing package.

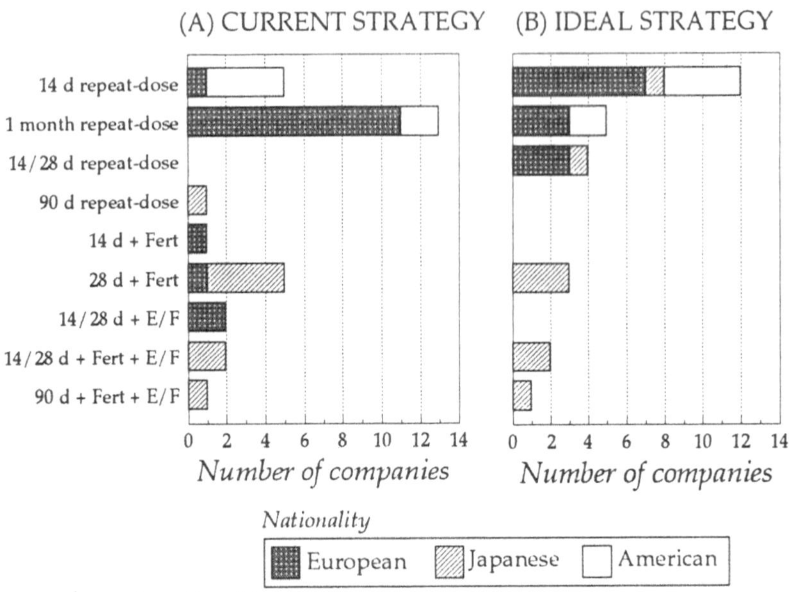

E/F = Embryo/foetal developmental toxicity study
Fert = Fertility study
PP = Pre- and post-natal developmental toxicity study

Figure 3.7 Reproductive and developmental toxicity studies conducted as part of current (A) or ideal (B) toxicity testing strategy to support the first administration of a new medicine to women of childbearing potential

In general, the range of suggested ideal strategies was broadly similar to the range of current approaches (Figure 3.7B). Three companies, however, considered that, initially, no reproductive studies would be necessary but qualified this by saying that the female subjects must be proven to be non-pregnant and covered by adequate contraceptive measures. The ideal approach to this issue was divergent between those who would conduct an embryo/foetal study as a maximum and those who would conduct fertility studies together with an embryo/foetal study as a minimum.

Ideal strategies

A summary of the ideal strategies for the three aspects of clinical development which were the subject of this initial investigation is shown in Table 3.2.

Table 3.2 Summary of favoured ideal approaches to the timing of toxicity studies suggested by survey participants

Clinical stage	*Completed supporting toxicity studies*
The first administration of a new medicine to humans	• Bacterial mutation test plus one or two tests for chromosome damage • Acute toxicity • 14-day repeated dose toxicity
Repeated dosing in humans	• 1- or 3-month toxicity studies to support up to one month clinical use • 6-month toxicity studies to support up to six months clinical use
The first inclusion of women of child-bearing potential in clinical trials	• Genetic toxicology • Acute toxicology • Repeated dose toxicology • (i) Maximum of embryo/foetal developmental toxicity ***or*** (ii) minimum of female fertility plus embryo/foetal developmental toxicity

Discussion and conclusions

Harmonising the differences between European, American and Japanese guidelines on the toxicity studies required to support the various stages of clinical development should serve two purposes. The first would be to eliminate any redundant testing in animals being carried out purely to satisfy country-specific regulatory requirements, the second would be to improve the efficiency of the developmental process by encouraging the use of single international strategies. For ethical considerations, the first of these is reason enough to argue for harmonisation. Regarding improvements in efficiency, toxicity testing tends to be most frequently rate limiting before clinical trials are initiated. Therefore, any savings in time and resources will generally be the result of streamlining preclinical development prior to the initial clinical investigations in humans. If this is to be achieved, attention should be focused towards reaching a consensus on the *minimum* acceptable preclinical package.

Two areas of the timing of toxicity testing that stand out as having diverse scientific approaches are the reproductive studies carried out before including women in clinical trials and the need for carcinogenicity tests to support Phase III. These animal studies are particularly important in the planning of an effective timing strategy because of their large use of time and resources. The relevance of the animal data for the clinical use, at whatever stage of development, should always be borne in mind. The questions that have been raised on the utility of carcinogenicity testing (Monro, 1993) are therefore important and have a place in the timing debate. Similarly, strong scientific principles need to be attached to the suggestions for reproductive and developmental toxicity studies to support the use of women in clinical trials, especially since the new Food and Drug Administration (FDA) "gender" guideline (FDA, 1993) serves to encourage the earlier involvement of women in clinical development. Reproductive toxicity tests should not be brought earlier into the testing strategy purely to provide "comfort factors".

There is much variation in the approach by companies to the timing of toxicity studies in relation to clinical investigation. Although some of this may be due to differences in the regulatory authorities' guidelines between the three regions, the responses to questions concerning an ideal, *unregulated* approach clearly demonstrate that this variation is also due to differences in scientific and strategic thinking. Any consensus reached regarding suggestions for an international guideline will need to resolve extreme differences in scientific thinking but also must provide sufficient flexibility for the different strategic needs of individual companies developing different types of compounds. This survey, of which some preliminary results have been presented here, will provide a baseline from which a consensus may develop.

References

Monro A (1993). How useful are chronic (life-span) toxicology studies in rodents in identifying pharmaceuticals that pose a carcinogenic risk to humans? *Adverse Drug Reactions and Toxicological Reviews*, **12**: 5–34.

Scales MDC and Mahoney K (1991). Animal toxicology studies on new medicines and their relationship to clinical exposure: a review of international recommendations. *Adverse Drug Reactions and Toxicological Reviews*, **10**: 155–168.

FDA, Department of Health and Human Services (1993). Guideline for the study and evaluation of gender differences in the clinical evaluation of drugs. *Federal Register*, **58 (139)**: 39406–39416.

4 Considerations for implementing a toxicity testing strategy

DOUGLAS M MORTON

Summary

1. All potential new drugs should be adequately tested in a series of widely accepted and well proven toxicological studies prior to first administration to humans. The study design should be scientifically credible and meet current worldwide government regulatory requirements.
2. The test compound, although in limited supply at an early stage of development, should meet scientifically acceptable analytical standards. The test compound used in the subchronic and chronic studies should closely resemble that to be used in the pivotal clinical trials and future marketing.
3. Selection of the most relevant species for the toxicity studies should be based on an early knowledge of the absorption and metabolism of the compound in the animal species and comparisons to data obtained in humans.
4. Incorporation of quality assessments into all parts of a testing programme can prevent the need for costly and time-consuming repeat studies and can preserve an efficient drug development programme.

Introduction

In a rapidly changing pharmaceutical industry, there is an important need for efficient new drug development. Decisions must be made at the earliest opportunity to determine whether the new compound is efficacious and safe or whether the project should be discontinued, with the redirection or saving of important resources. Thus, the creation of a plan for efficient and rational toxicological testing, an integral part of the new drug development process, is vital. One approach will be presented here.

Strategy for study design

The incorporation of the best scientific principles into the animal toxicology and supporting absorption, distribution, metabolism, and excretion (ADME) studies is essential. The programme should also be designed to meet current worldwide regulatory guidelines to permit successful drug approval and registration. Initial toxicological studies should be based on a knowledge of the proposed clinical dosing plan; clinical pharmacology in human volunteers and efficacy studies in patients including route of administration, projected dosage range and regimen, duration of dosing, and the geographical location where the initial studies will be performed. The subsequent clinical efficacy and safety studies in patients will be based on the data from the clinical pharmacology studies. An example of a typical development plan is shown in Figure 4.1.

The pilot toxicity studies will often include acute toxicity determinations in rats and mice, mutagenicity studies (such as Ames bacterial test and an *in vivo* rat micronucleus assay), expanded general pharmacology studies, and 7- to 14-day repeat-dose studies in rodents and non-rodents. Data can be obtained on possible liver enzyme induction at the end of the repeated dose period and bone marrow cells from the rats can be examined for the presence of micronuclei to confirm findings in the pilot mutagenicity studies. The pilot tests may be performed on a single approved project compound or on a series of compounds from discovery research for which a final selection is still needed. The data may or may not be used to support initial clinical testing in human volunteers; if it is to be used, the toxicity tests and supporting ADME studies should be performed under good laboratory practice (GLP) regulations.

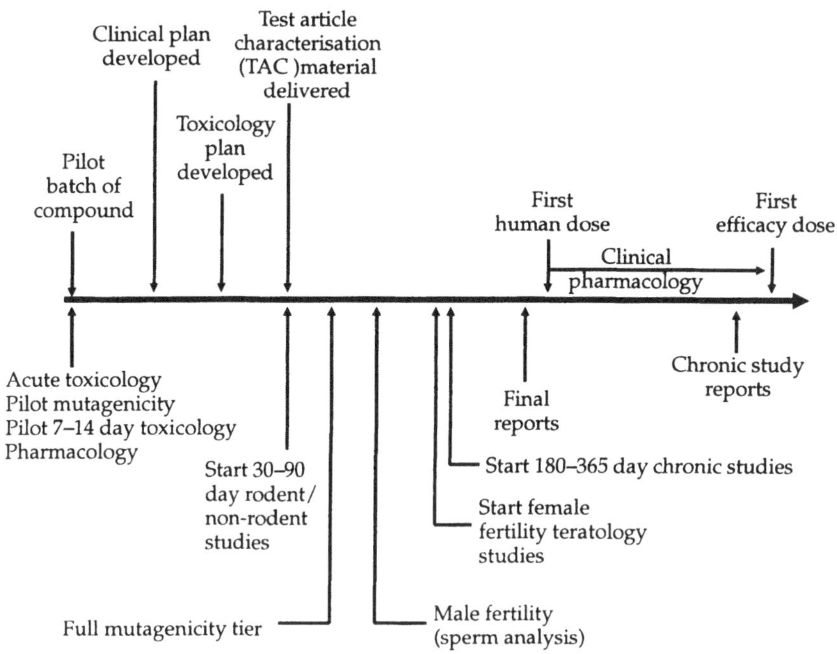

Figure 4.1 Development plan for toxicity studies

Subchronic toxicity studies of 14 days' duration in a rodent and non-rodent species can normally support a single dose in healthy volunteers or three single doses during a one-week period.

Test compounds should meet acceptable analytical and purity standards using validated testing methods as shown in Table 4.1. Every effort should be made to limit the presence of residual solvents, heavy metals, or other impurities resulting from the synthetic processes. However, it is recognised that at this early stage of development, quantities of the new compound are often limited; the compound has usually been synthesised by a "less than optimal" synthetic route and the analytical purity may not meet the requirements of a final marketed drug. Data demonstrating stability of the test compound under acid conditions should be a prerequisite for compounds to be orally administered.

In many cases the pilot studies are used to help design subsequent definitive toxicity studies. Where possible, the same synthetic batch of the new compound should be used for these definitive studies and the early clinical trials; the batch of material should meet stringent analytical standards in the test article characterisation (TAC) (Table 4.1). In addition, compounds for human clinical trials in the USA should be synthesised under good manufacturing practices (GMP).

Table 4.1 Analytical testing of new compounds

For pilot toxicity studies:	*For definitive toxicity studies Test article characterisation (TAC):*
Elemental analysis (C,H,N)	Assays as for pilot studies plus:
Identity (IR, UV, mass spectroscopy)	Potency
NMR	Purity
Melting point	HPLC assay
Solubility	Related substances
Acid/base stability	Other impurities including solvents and heavy metals
	X-ray diffraction
	Dose form, stability data

Toxicological support for clinical studies

Administration of single doses to human volunteers can provide early information on pharmacology and possible adverse side-effects together with data on human oral absorption, plasma levels, plasma half-life, and route of excretion. However, such data are often insufficient to make a final decision on the development of the new drug. More often, the testing proceeds as quickly as possible to multiple doses in volunteers and studies in patients (Phase IB or Phase II clinical studies). Thus, 30-day subchronic toxicity studies in a rodent and non-rodent species are usually performed immediately after the pilot studies. Data from these tests can support dosing in patients for up to one week in Europe and up to 30 days in the USA, the latter following submission and approval of an investigational new drug application (IND). To support early efficacy studies in humans of greater than 30 days, the completion of 90- or 180-day toxicity studies will be necessary. All of these subchronic or chronic studies should be performed under GLP guidelines using compound for which a test article characterisation has been completed.

To support absorption and bioavailability studies in laboratory animals and humans, a sensitive and accurate analytical method for the compound in plasma and urine should be developed at an early stage (Figure 4.2). In addition, the synthesis of radio-labelled compound can significantly aid studies on absorption and tissue distribution using whole body autoradiography, metabolism, and excretion. Such data can assist in the selection of relevant laboratory species for the toxicity studies and subsequent comparisons with data obtained in humans. Early information on the comparative metabolism of the compound can be obtained by incubating the test compound with liver microsomal preparations from animals and humans (Figure 4.3).

At this stage of development, and prior to repeated dosage in humans, a full tier of widely used and accepted mutagenicity studies should be completed with the TAC compound (Table 4.2).

Studies should also be performed to ensure that the new compound does not produce adverse effects on male fertility. Such information can be obtained by careful histopathological examination of the male reproductive organs in the species used for the 30-day subchronic studies together with a 14-day study in rats to examine possible effects on the structure and motility of the rat

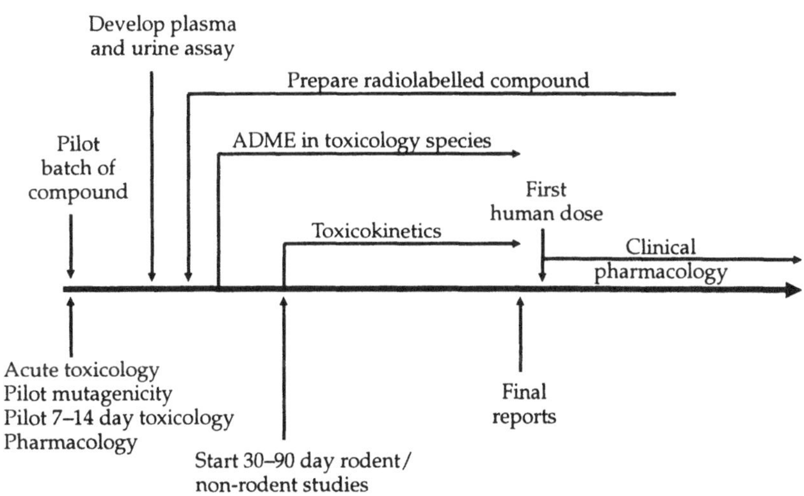

Figure 4.2 Development plan for ADME studies

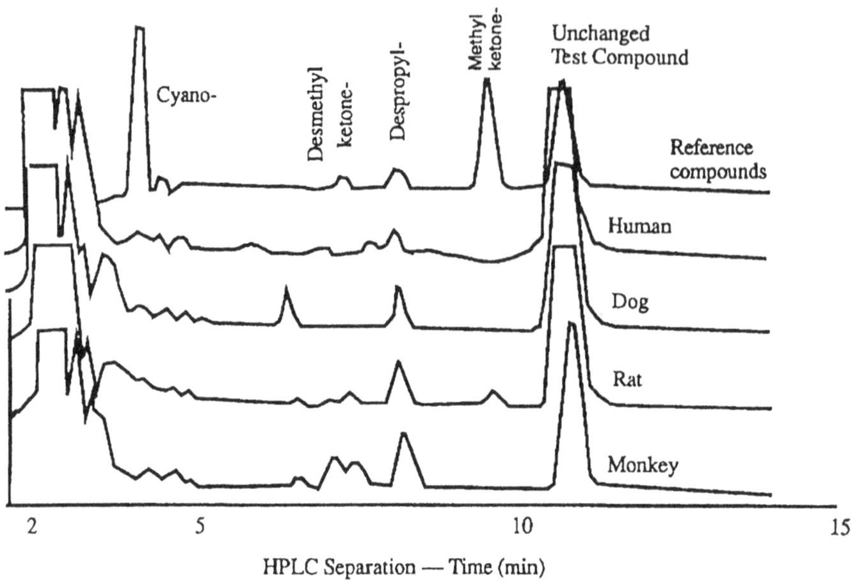

Figure 4.3 Comparative metabolism with liver microsomal preparations

Table 4.2 Tier of mutagenicity studies

Pilot studies
Gradient plate bacterial assay
Pilot *in vivo* mirconucleus test (14-day rat study)
Definitive studies (TAC compound)
Ames plate assay
Mouse lymphoma assay
In vitro chromosome aberration test (CHO cells)
In vivo micronucleus test in rats

sperm. The design for the latter study is shown in Figure 4.4. If women of childbearing potential are to be included in the volunteer studies or early patient studies, teratology studies should be completed in rats and rabbits together with a determination of possible adverse effects in rats on female fertility. As in the subchronic toxicity studies, bioavailability of the test compound should be proven in the pregnant rats or rabbits together with evidence of exposure of the

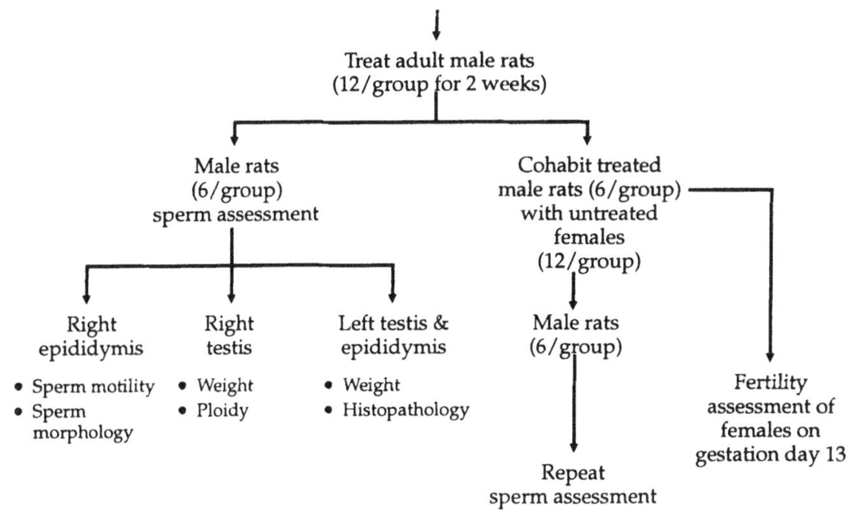

Figure 4.4 Design for study of spermatogenesis, sperm quality, and reproductive performance in rats. Adapted from Hoyt *et al.* (1994)

foetus. Foetal exposure should be determined by autoradiographic studies on pregnant animals during the important period of organogenesis or by direct chemical analysis of extracts of foetal tissues.

With the assumption that the new compound has shown acceptable bioavailability in the human volunteers and has not produced unacceptable adverse side-effects, chronic toxicity studies, to support longer term (Phase III) studies in patients, and eventual drug registration, should be initiated at this stage. The length of the chronic studies in rodents and non-rodents will be dependent on the duration of the proposed clinical testing and the future therapeutic regimens. In general, these tests are of six months duration in rodents and six to 12 months in dogs or monkeys. To ensure an efficient and uninterrupted clinical programme, these studies should be commenced soon after the completion of the first human dose and clinical pharmacology (Figure 4.1); the selection of doses being based on the data from the 30-day tests. The batch of compound used should meet the requirements of the TAC, be the most suitable salt form, where applicable be in the most stable crystalline form, and of a particle size to permit maximal bioavailability. This batch of compound should also be analytically representative of the material to be used in the Phase III clinical trials and subsequent marketing.

Throughout all of these toxicity and ADME studies, the protocol design, study performance, collection of all experimental data, and preparation of the final reports should be of the highest possible quality. The continual evaluation of quality indicators (Figure 4.5) should be an integral part of all studies to ensure that accuracy is not compromised and efficiency is maintained throughout the development of the drug. A comprehensive quality control programme established in each of the laboratories conducting the toxicology and ADME studies can markedly improve the quality of the data and limit the necessity for detailed quality assurance reviews.

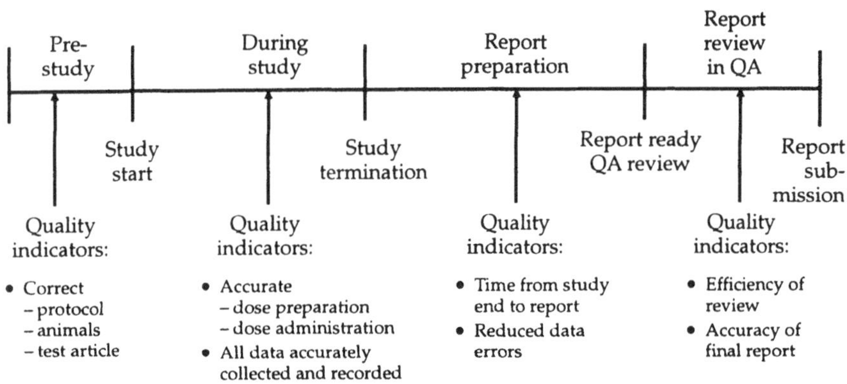

Figure 4.5 Quality indicators in toxicity studies

Conclusion

The toxicological studies designed to support the clinical evaluation of a new drug should be scientifically credible and meet the requirements and recommendations of worldwide regulatory agencies. The quality of the test compound, although undergoing continual improvement during the development process, should meet high standards. The selection of the most relevant species for the toxicity studies should be based on a detailed knowledge of the absorption, distribution, and metabolism of the test compound and comparisons to *in vitro* and *in vivo* data obtained from humans. The incorporation of quality assessments (quality control and quality assurance) into all parts of a valid testing programme can prevent the need for costly and time-consuming repeat studies and can preserve an efficient drug development programme.

References

Hoyt JA, Fisher LF, Hoffman WP, Swisher DK and Seyler DE (1994). Utilisation of a short-term male reproductive toxicity study design to examine effects of α-chlorohydrin (3-chloro-1,2-propanediol). *Reproductive Toxicology*, **8**,(3), 237–250

SECTION II

Personal Views

5 Phase I clinical trials: what is the minimum preclinical package necessary for initiating single-dose studies in man? – a toxicologist's opinion

HERMAN VAN CAUTEREN

Summary

1. To achieve harmonisation of the requirements for toxicity testing to support the initiation of single-dose studies in man between Europe, the USA and Japan, more emphasis should be placed on the scientific rationale as presented in the safety assessment document (SAD). The SAD contains a summary of the preclinical findings, with a discussion of their clinical relevance, including a quantitative and qualitative assessment.
2. The normal set of toxicity studies for a single-dose Phase I study in humans consists of: single-dose toxicity studies in two animal species using one or two routes of administration; repeated dose toxicity studies in two species using the clinical route of administration and lasting two to four weeks; and two mutagenicity studies, usually an *in vitro* Ames test and an *in vivo* micronucleus test.
3. Harmonisation should focus on a flexible, safety-based approach. In addition to optimal compliance with the scientific, regulatory and legal aspects for initiating the first clinical trials in man, ethical considerations are important for both human exposure and laboratory animal use.

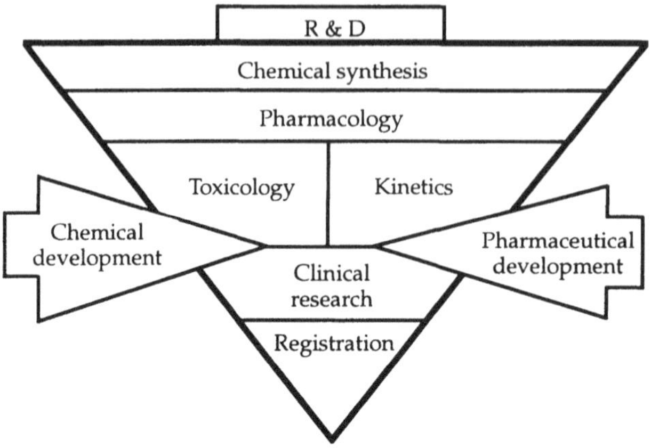

Figure 5.1 Pharmaceutical R & D activities

The Safety Assessment Document

It is proposed that the minimum preclinical package necessary for the initiation of single-dose studies in man should be in the form of the "Safety Assessment Document (SAD)". This short document contains a summary of the preclinical findings with a discussion of their clinical relevance, including a quantitative (safety margin and systemic exposure) and qualitative assessment giving insight into the nature of the findings and their proposed pathogenesis. The SAD concept originates from the Nordic guidelines. The Swedish authorities have published their recommendations on pharmacological and toxicological documentation (Anon, 1983). With regard to the safety assessment, these guidelines state that *"a summarised evaluation and safety assessment with relation to the proposed clinical trials must be included in the light of the extent and results of the pharmacological and toxicological studies carried out"*.

Included in the preclinical package are chemical, pharmaceutical, pharmacodynamic, pharmacokinetic and toxicological development activities (Figure 5.1).

Chemical development

During early chemical development, synthesis of the first chemical batch and its analytical assessment takes place. Since this comprises the early stage of the development, good manufacturing practice (GMP) compliance can be minimal. Ideally, one chemical batch of appropriate quality should be used for preclinical as well as clinical studies. The advantage of using the same batch in both types of studies is that the impurity content is comparable. If more than one batch is used, batch purities should be compared. Mutagenicity studies should be done with the batch that will be used in clinical trials.

Pharmaceutical development

Pharmaceutical development should provide sufficient information and documentation on the composition of the formulation and mode of administration for use in animals and, if applicable, in man. Solutions are preferred for oral dosing in order to maximise oral bioavailability in both animals and man. Relatively non-toxic, solubilising agents such as cyclodextrins (e.g. hydroxypropyl-β-cyclodextrin) may be useful for new pharmaceuticals with a low water solubility (Mesens *et al.*, 1991; Mesens *et al.*, 1992). Adherence to minimal GMP standards is a requirement. According to the duration of intended use, the formulation should be subjected to the appropriate stability testing.

Pharmacodynamics

The primary and secondary pharmacodynamic effects are studied in a limited number of animal models. The primary pharmacodynamics of a new candidate pharmaceutical are investigated in studies conducted *in vitro* and *in vivo*. These studies should provide evidence for specificity and selectivity of the main activity of the pharmaceutical. Evaluation of the secondary *in vitro* and *in vivo* pharmacodynamics is equally important to identify potential effects not associated with the main activity. Of particular importance are findings affecting vital functions including central nervous system, cardiovascular and pulmonary functions.

This evaluation should, preferably, be done at the anticipated therapeutic and at supra-therapeutic dose levels. If possible, the formulation (e.g. an oral solution) intended for clinical trials should be used. These studies should be of a high quality and the decision as to whether they should be carried out according to good laboratory practice or not (they can be either safety or pharmacology studies) should be made by the individual pharmaceutical company.

Pharmacokinetics

Validated and sensitive methodology to measure active drug concentrations in body fluids and organs is a prerequisite for conducting pharmacokinetic studies (Heykants and Meuldermans, 1993). The first single-dose pharmacokinetic measurements are often done in pharmacodynamic studies. Hereby, pharmacodynamic studies are validated for systemic exposure. Findings from these studies also supply early information on issues such as dose-linearity, interspecies differences in absorption, metabolism or excretion. Repeated dose pharmacokinetic measurements are usually done in conjunction with the repeated dose toxicity studies. Hereby, not only plasma levels but also levels in several potentially important target tissues are measured, although the latter measurement should not be considered an absolute necessity at this early stage of development. Not only *in vivo* pharmacokinetic studies but also *in vitro* studies are often conducted concurrently. These studies make use of hepatic microsomal fractions derived from some of the main laboratory animal species (rat, dog) and from humans. In some cases, studies using primary hepatocyte cultures from various species can also provide useful information. Working with cell cultures offers the advantages that the pharmacometabolism resembles the *in vivo* situation and cytotoxicity can be included as an endpoint parameter.

Toxicology

The normal set of toxicity studies for a single-dose Phase I study in humans consists of:

1. Single-dose toxicity studies in two animal species using one or two routes of administration. Currently, rats and mice are the

mammalian species of choice (according to the First International Conference on Harmonisation (ICH1) (D'Arcy and Harron, 1991)). The chosen route of administration in these studies depends on the intended route of administration in clinical trials.

If the proposed clinical route is parenteral (usually intravenous (iv)) then it is sufficient to conduct toxicology using the parenteral route only. If the proposed clinical route is oral, then studies using both oral and iv routes are conducted. The fixed-dose procedure or any other dosing regimen resulting in a minimum number of dose levels are used for these single-dose studies.

2. Repeated dose toxicity studies in two species using the clinical route of administration and lasting two to four weeks.

   Amongst the rodent and non-rodent species required for this type of study, rats and dogs are the animals of choice. The proposed clinical route of administration is also used in the animal studies. Studies are conducted for a period of two to four weeks using, preferably, the formulation intended for clinical trials. As already mentioned, formulations which can be administered as oral solutions are given preference. A study duration of two weeks suffices for a single-dose protocol in human volunteers. If one plans to continue thereafter with a repeated dose protocol in clinical trials, the duration of the toxicity studies should preferably be four weeks.

3. Two mutagenicity studies, being usually an *in vitro* Ames test and an *in vivo* micronucleus test.

   The Ames test is used for detection of gene and point mutations. The micronucleus test in mice or rats is considered to be an appropriate *in vivo* test to detect chromosome aberrations. With reference to ICH2, dose level selection in this test should be validated according to endpoints of toxicity or systemic exposure (D'Arcy and Harron, 1994). An alternative to the micronucleus test is the *in vitro* chromosome aberration test in human lymphocytes. However, an *in vivo* test is preferred to *in vitro* testing.

If a second systemic route of administration is to be used in humans, the available set of toxicity studies is complemented by repeat-dose toxicity studies in two species using the second route of administration. When the second clinical route is topical, a single-dose topical irritation study should be conducted, and for compounds for which systemic exposure is not intended to be present, pharmacokinetic evidence for this must be generated.

Comparison between the three regions (the European Community, the USA and Japan)

When the requirements for toxicity testing in the three defined regions are compared, it is apparent that the European Community is the least demanding. Either a local (i.e. Ethical Committee) or a national application for clinical trials can be made, usually a 2-week repeated dose toxicity study suffices and no specific fertility study is required.

The authorities in the USA request a national application. Male fertility studies are not obligatory at this stage and American authorities are more flexible in their requirements concerning the duration of animal toxicity studies which should precede clinical trials.

The situation in Japan is somewhat more demanding since like the USA only a national application is possible; however, the minimum requirement is a 1-month repeat dose study as well as a male fertility study in rats for conducting trials with male volunteers.

Future harmonisation

For further harmonisation of these requirements, more emphasis should be placed on the scientific rationale as presented in the SAD. This includes an appropriate estimation of the degree of risk involved. In this sense, this view fits well with the probability discussion on the degree of risk as put forward by Günzel and Bass (1991) (Figure 5.2).

Depending on the conclusions derived from the SAD, the option exists to either perform additional preclinical studies or to initiate clinical trials with the available set of information. It is therefore important to clearly distinguish between the requirements for an open, dose-escalating Phase I study in healthy human volunteers, a Phase II and a Phase III study in patients. The degree of risk involved is different and, because of this, a file for clinical research is not the same as a registration file for marketing application. In this respect, it is interesting to note that the authorities from the three regions

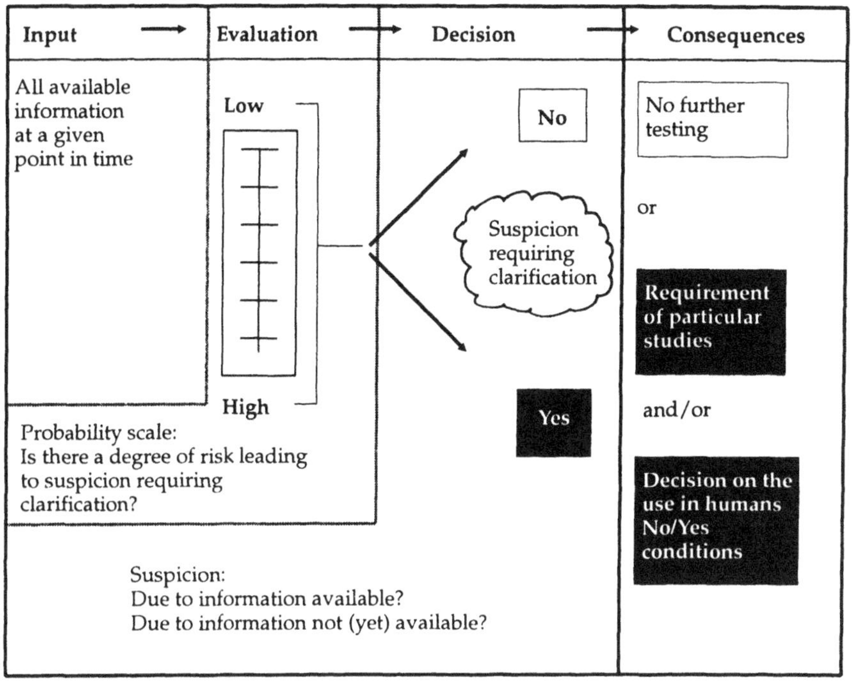

Figure 5.2 Considerations regarding the development of individual non-clinical test strategies in the European Community (Reproduced from Günzel and Bass (1991) with permission).

currently adopt a more flexible attitude to the former. A typical example of this is given in a recent EC directive for testing of medicinal products, (91/507/EEC Annex, part 3, chapter II,A,2 on repeated dose toxicity). Of particular interest is the last sentence of this quotation when considering its application for the ICH process:

"Generally, it is desirable that two tests be performed: one short-term, lasting two to four weeks, the other long-term. The duration of the latter shall depend on the conditions of clinical use. Its purpose shall be to determine by experiment the non-toxic dose range of the product and normally it shall last three to six months.

In respect of medicinal products to be administered once only to humans, a single test lasting two to four weeks shall be performed.

If, however, having regarded the proposed duration of use in human beings, the investigator sees fit to carry out experiments of greater or lesser duration than indicated above, he must give adequate reasons for doing so."

In a nutshell, harmonisation should be mainly based upon a safety-based flexibility. In addition to optimal compliance with the scientific, regulatory and legal aspects for initiating the first clinical trials in man, ethical considerations are important for both human exposure and laboratory animal use. In this respect, harmonisation will also contribute to the three "Rs" (Reduction, Refinement, Replacement) concerning the use of laboratory animals.

Acknowledgements

The author wishes to thank Johanna Benze, Werner Coussement, Ann Lampo, John Vandenberghe and Philippe Vanparys for their helpful comments.

References

Anon (1983). Swedish Instructions and General Guidelines on Clinical Trials of Drugs, November 22, 1983.

D'Arcy PF and Harron DWG (eds) (1991). *Proceedings of The First International Conference on Harmonisation, Brussels, 1991.* The Queen's University of Belfast.

D'Arcy PF and Harron DWG (eds) (1994). *Proceedings of The Second International Conference on Harmonisation, Orlando, USA 1993.* The Queen's University of Belfast (in press).

Günzel P and Bass R (1991). Considerations regarding the development of individual nonclinical test strategies in the European Community. *Human & Experimental Toxicology*, **10**, 297–304.

Heykants J and Meuldermans W (1993). Nonclinical kinetics and metabolism studies in support of the safety assessment of drugs. *Drug Information Journal*, **28**, 163–172.

Mesens JL, Putteman P and Verheyen P (1991). Pharmaceutical applications of 2-hydroxypropyl-β-cyclodextrin: preclinical studies and current clinical developments. In: Duchêne D (ed.) *Editions de Santé*, Paris, France, September 1991.

Mesens JL, Meuldermans W, Szathmary S and Putteman P (1992). In vivo behavior of the drug-cyclodextrin complex: supermolecule or just a complex. *Abstracts of the Sixth International Cyclodextrin Symposium, Chicago, April 1992.*

6 Phase I clinical trials: what is the minimum preclinical package necessary for initiating single-dose studies in man? – a clinical pharmacologist's opinion

DIANE JORKASKY

Summary

1. There seems to be no clear scientific rationale underpinning the guideline that states that two species, one of which is a non-rodent, need to be treated for two weeks to allow single dosing in humans. This does not take into account the properties of the drug being tested, the indication, the risks versus benefits of the drug or the target population.
2. The toxicology package that is currently used to support the initiation of single-dose studies in humans appears to be fairly adequate in that rarely does the development of a compound stop in early Phase I due to safety reasons.
3. The following concerns should be addressed prior to dosing humans with a new chemical entity for the first time: safety pharmacology of major end organs (CNS, CVS/renal, pulmonary); causes of death in animals; genotoxicity; preliminary evaluation of the metabolic profile, dosing long enough in animals to ensure that the duration of a single-dose exposure in humans is covered; and an assessment of toxicokinetics.

Introduction

This is a difficult topic to address because companies tend to think about what is needed to support the fastest development of a new chemical entity to a GO/NO GO decision point rather than to a single dose in humans. Rarely is the first study in humans going to provide adequate information to stop the further development of a drug. Most companies do not find themselves with the luxury of being able to simultaneously introduce several compounds of the same pharmacological type into humans to determine the best candidate. It is with this perspective that the question has been approached.

The problem

There seems to be no clear scientific rationale underpinning the guideline that states that two species, one of which is a non-rodent, need to be treated for two weeks to allow single dosing in humans. Unfortunately the guideline has become the standard, a standard which does not take into account the properties of the drug being tested, the indication, the risks versus benefits of the drug, or the target population. Only with drugs to be used in oncology and in the treatment of AIDS does some flexibility appear.

The science of the toxicological evaluation of a drug to be used for single dosing should rely upon:

- the known pharmacology of the drug;
- the known chemical nature of the drug;
- the kinetics of the drug as they are known from animal studies and to what they may be reasonably extrapolated in humans;
- an assessment of the data generated in animal pharmacology models; and
- a good understanding of toxicological "history".

There are a great deal of data on the effects of various chemical classes of drugs in laboratory animals that probably have been forgotten or, unfortunately, never published, that may be able to help both the toxicologist and the clinical pharmacologist make better informed decisions. Moreover, the toxicological programme should also consider how the drug will be delivered to humans, what will be the duration of administration, and the population into whom it is being introduced. For example, cancer chemotherapeutic agents may have profound toxicity in animals, but these do not negate proceeding into humans. What purpose then do extensive pathological and toxicological studies serve with this class of agent? Similarly, if a drug is targeted for a rapidly fatal disease, and this is the patient population to whom the drug will first be administered, one could argue for a minimal toxicological evaluation.

The "art" of toxicology comes to bear in compiling appropriate studies that address these issues and in interpreting the relevance of the data derived from those studies to humans.

The specific requirements of a preclinical data package depends to some extent upon the philosophy regarding Phase I testing. The use of normal volunteers or patients with the disease will influence this. In dealing with normal volunteers, does one take the dose to the point of "toxicity" or to some comfortable level and allow toxicity to be expressed in patients where one could argue that benefit clearly outweighs risk? Volunteers should be dosed to a level that puts them in no harm, yet addresses the issue of pharmacology and toxicology as much as possible. What this level is depends upon the drug and specifically its known pharmacology and potential toxicity. On occasion, guidance from pharmacological endpoints, for example, Q-T interval prolongation with an antiarrhythmic or by direct observation of signs or symptoms, can be used. Particular attention needs to be paid to evaluating those markers of end organ damage that have been identified in toxicological testing or from known effects from drugs of a similar class that have already been in humans. The relatively weak relationship between animal toxicity and human toxicity is well recognised, so it is important not to ignore signs of other end organs that were not implicated in toxicological studies. Often the top dose may be reached due to some physical limitation in the compound's administration, for example, volunteers having to ingest large quantities of fairly unpalatable liquid or a large number of tablets. The top dose level used in subjects will, in the end, largely be determined by using good clinical judgement.

Minimum preclinical package

What does the clinical pharmacologist want as the minimum preclinical package necessary for initiating single-dose studies in humans? The toxicology packages used to date seem to be fairly adequate in that rarely does the development of a compound stop in early Phase I due to safety reasons. If this is the experience throughout the industry, then why should the current situation be changed?

A single dose of a drug, even if found to be toxic in long-term studies, is unlikely to be harmful if given to humans in a slow dose-ascendancy trial. Thus, what clinical pharmacologists really want to know is how toxic a drug is when given to animals in a few doses. From these studies, some estimate of the dose (or pharmacokinetic) margins between no effect and significant toxicity should be provided.

One reason for the apparent lack of relationship between toxicity in humans and animals may be the historical dependence upon dose/toxicity relationships. Only in the last few years has there been greater use of evaluating toxicity with pharmacokinetic parameters of the drug. This seems to be an approach that may still be underutilised in evaluating drug toxicity. Toxicokinetic evaluation may be worth scrutinising as an approach to improve the predictability of animal pathology/toxicology for human toxicity. Refinement of pharmacokinetic/ pharmacodynamic modelling may reveal relationships between certain kinetic parameters and toxicity that are not apparent on the basis of dose. There are several examples in the literature where such modelling is not only helpful in evaluating toxicity but in demonstrating pharmacological comparability of the animal data to humans. Perhaps it may then be possible to extract more valuable data from fewer animals.

In summary, a list of the clinical pharmacologists' concerns which need to be addressed prior to dosing humans with a "routine" new chemical entity for the first time is given in Table 1.

Harmonisation has made us all re-evaluate practices that seemed to be so antiquated, they were etched in stone. Perhaps it is time to break the tablets.

Table 6.1 Concerns that need to be addressed prior to the first dose of an NCE in man

Safety assessment required for first compound into man	*Comment*
Safety pharmacology of major end organs in unanaesthetised animals: CNS, cardiovascular/renal, pulmonary	These studies parallel more closely the endpoints utilised in the evaluation of volunteers or patients in human studies in Phase I.
Assessment of pharmacology "run amok" versus true *de novo* toxicity	
Understanding of causes of death in animals	
Genotoxicity (Ames, mouse lymphoma, etc.)	There is an ethical obligation to advise the volunteer/patient of such potential.
Preliminary evaluation of the metabolic profile, specifically, site(s) of elimination, metabolism, etc.	This information is particularly helpful with drugs that may have active metabolites with long half- lives.
Dosing long enough in animals to make sure that the duration of a single-dose exposure in human is covered	For drugs with a short half-life, 5–7 day dosing in dogs and two weeks dosing in rodents is probably adequate. For drugs with very long half-lives, study duration should be extended beyond two weeks to cover the interval. For example, two weeks dosing with a drug that has an 18-day half-life requires that the animal be monitored beyond the dosing period for the development of toxicity.
Assessment of toxicokinetics	It is important to understand whether the drug was absorbed, and how toxicity may be related to the various kinetic parameters (*AUC* C_{max}, etc.) in addition to dose. Continued evaluation of this approach, in addition to dose/toxicity response, may be helpful in allowing better correlation between human and animal data. Further refinement of kinetic/dynamic modelling approaches may be helpful.

7 The duration of toxicity studies required to support repeated dosing in clinical investigation – a toxicologist's opinion

TOSHIJI IGARASHI

Summary

1. Animal data are essential for the safety assessment of new drugs, particularly when initiating clinical trials where little or no human data are available. However, the duration of toxicity studies required to support repeated dosing in humans should be discussed on a more scientific basis, taking into consideration the relationship between the duration of repeated dosing and new toxicity findings in animals, the reliability of the results of animal studies at predicting potential safety in clinical use, and the relationship of the time-scale in different animal species to man.
2. It is proposed that four weeks repeated dosing in animals is sufficient to support studies in humans up to four weeks. Following this, 3-month repeated dose toxicity studies should be recommended as the minimum duration to support repeated dosing of longer than four weeks in all phases of clinical investigation.
3. Long-term dosing in humans, such as that over six months, can only be supported by human data which are accumulated by the step-wise process of clinical investigation.

Duration of repeated dosing and new toxicity findings

For repeated dosing in clinical trials of up to four weeks in humans, the authorities in the USA, the EC and Japan unanimously recommend 13 weeks repeated dose toxicity testing in animals. The questions that needs to be answered are: what is the scientific basis of these recommendations and what is the rationale for recommending 6-month repeated dose toxicity studies to support clinical trials of longer than four weeks? There are three aspects that need to be considered in addressing these questions: (i) what is the relationship between the duration of repeated dosing and new toxicity findings in animals; (ii) how reliable are the results of animal studies at predicting potential safety in clinical use; and (iii) how does the time-scale in different animal species relate to that in man?

Relationship between duration and new toxicity findings

Several detailed studies have investigated the relationship between the duration of repeated dosing and new toxicity findings (e.g. Contrera *et al.*, 1993, Igarashi, 1992, Igarashi, 1993, Lumley *et al.*, 1993). One of these compared the No Observed Effect Levels (NOEL) and toxicity findings in 114 paired 3- and 12-month studies in rats, dogs or monkeys conducted in Japan within the past seven years. There were no definite quantitative differences between the 3- and 12-month studies, and the results demonstrated that most toxicities could be identified within three months (Igarashi, 1992). Similarly, there were no distinct differences in the toxicity findings of paired 6- and 12-month studies in dogs, examined in databases established by the Japanese Pharmaceutical Manufacturers' Association (JPMA) (Igarashi, 1993), the Centre for Medicines Research (CMR) (Lumley *et al.*, 1993) and the US Food and Drug Administration (FDA) (Contrera *et al.*, 1993).

The improvement in the design of toxicological studies is more important than the length of dosing beyond three or six months. In a second JPMA study, four of the 90 cases examined revealed new toxicities at 12 months that were not detectable during the first three months of the study. However, in one of these, abnormal ossification caused by a bone calcium regulator was not related to the length of exposure but to the timing (the stage of skeletal growth and development) of exposure. In a second, gingival hypertrophy caused by

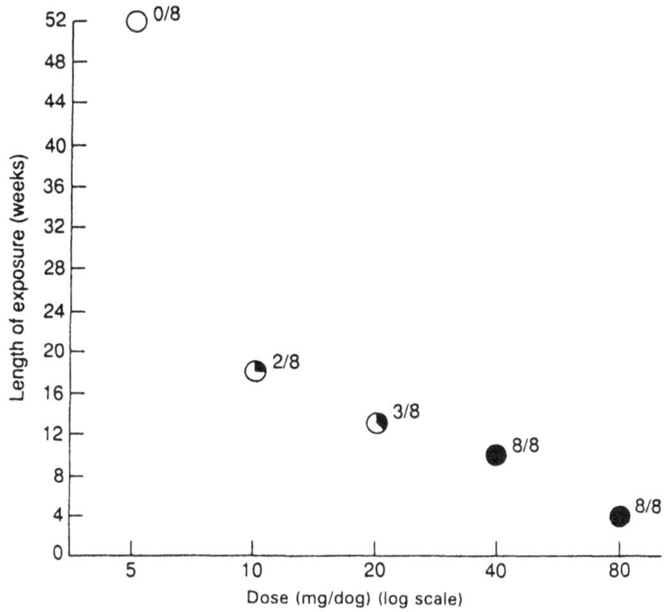

Figure 7.1 Test dose and time (weeks of exposure to a calcium antagonist) of onset of gingival hyperplasia in a 52-week study in dogs. *Figures beside symbols indicate proportion of animals with hyperplasia.* Reproduced from Igarashi (1993) by permission of Oxford University Press.

a calcium antagonist could be detected in week 4 of treatment, depending on the test dose (Figure 7.1). The gingival hyperplasia was not observed in a 52-week study in any of eight dogs treated with 5 mg/kg, but it developed in two of eight dogs treated with 10 mg/kg at the 18th week, in three dogs treated with 20 mg/kg at the 12th week, and in all eight animals treated at 40 or 80 mg/kg at the tenth and fourth weeks, respectively (Igarashi, 1993). An appropriate high dose selection in repeated dose toxicity studies therefore seems to be one of the key factors in shortening the period required to detect the toxicity of the test compound.

Predictability of adverse events by animal studies

In defining the appropriate duration of toxicity studies to support repeated dosing in clinical investigation, it is important to consider the extent to which animal data can be used to make reliable assessments of the safety of drugs for man, even excluding cases of idiosyncratic reactions and hypersensitivity. Two surveys have been conducted to address this question.

A literature survey of 139 drugs approved in Japan during 1987–1991

Over the past few years, a group within the JPMA has been investigating the reliability of animal studies in predicting clinical adverse events. A database created from the information in reports in Japanese journals has been used to assess the relationship between toxicities in animal studies and adverse events in clinical trials (JPMA, 1994). The survey investigations were repeated to check the consistency of the results, which showed a surprisingly poor relationship between specific toxicity in laboratory animals and adverse events in the clinic. For example, although measurement of alanine transaminase (ALT) and aspartate transaminase (AST) is commonly included in blood chemistry examinations in both animal toxicity studies and human clinical trials, there was no significant correlation between the human and animal data for the compounds examined (Table 7.1). However, closer examination of three case studies (Table 7.2) shows that the liver was identified as a target organ in all but one animal study, even though a specific effect on ALT or AST was not detected.

Table 7.1 Positive finding in animal studies for the increase in blood AST and/or ALT in the clinical trials

Rat studies	2/19
Dog studies	5/16
Monkey studies	2/5

A questionnaire survey of 64 New Chemical Entities (NCEs) withdrawn after IND due to safety problems during 1983–1992

A questionnaire-based survey was also carried out to obtain the animal data on drugs which were withdrawn from development due to adverse events observed in any phase of clinical development (JPMA, 1993). The results show that the relationship between the findings in animal studies and safety problems in the clinical is

Table 7.2 Case studies comparing hepatic effects in clinical trials with those in animal studies

Case A: Anti-hyperlipemic	
Clinical trial:	Early Phase II; 200–800 mg/day (p.o.) for 8 weeks increase in AST and ALT in 5/29 patients
Rat study:	30–3,000 mg/kg (p.o.) for 13 weeks increased liver organ weight, decreased plasma triglyceride (300 mg/kg), decreased plasma total cholersterol (3,000 mg/kg); but no case of increase of AST or ALT
Dog study:	30–1,000 mg/kg (p.o.) for 13 weeks decreased plasma total cholersterol (30 mg/kg), decreased plasma triglyceride, atrophy of hepatic cells, deposition of lipofuscin (100 mg/kg); increase in AST and ALT (100 mg/kg)
Case B: Antibiotic	
Clinical trial:	Phase I; single dose of 50–2,000 mg (iv) with a 2–3 weeks delay, increase in plasma AST, ALT alkaline phosphatase (ALP), lactate dehydrogenase (LDH), leucine aminopeptidase (LAP) and/or bilirubin in 4/12 treated with 1,000 or 2,000 mg/kg
Rat study:	50–450 mg/kg (iv) for 13 weeks no findings for the hepatic toxicity
Dog study:	50–450 mg/kg (iv) for 13 weeks increased hepatic organ weight and increased plasma total cholesterol (50 mg/kg); but no increase in AST or ALT or any related plasma enzyme activity
Case C: NSAID	
Clinical trial:	Phase I; single dose of 3–200 mg (p.o.), and repeated dose of 40 mg/day (p.o.) increased ALT and γ-glutamyl transferase (γ-GT) in 1/3 treated with single dose of 50 mg and 3/6 treated with 200 mg, and increased γ-GT, AST and/or ALT in 8/12 treated with a repeated dose of 40 mg/day for 21 days
Dog study:	1–250 mg/kg (p.o.) for 13 weeks increased hepatic organ weight and swelling of hepatic cells and smooth surfaced endoplasmic reticulum (50 mg/kg); but no increase in AST and ALT

Table 7.3 Classification of 91 adverse reactions found in 64 NCEs and relevance of the animal toxicity data to the clinical finding

		Relevance of animal data					
		Related		*Probably related*		*Not related*	
Safety problem	*No of clinical cases*	*Number*	*%*	*Number*	*%*	*Number*	*%*
Skin reactions	6	0	0	0	0	6	100
Psychological & nervous	9	2	22	5	55	2	22
Gastrointestinal	17	6	35	9	53	2	12
Hepatobilliary	29	2	7	9	31	18	62
Cardiovascular	7	6	86	0	0	1	14
Haematological	4	1	25	0	0	3	75
Others	19	5	31	7	44	7	44
Total	91	22	24	30	33	39	43

variable. Not surprisingly, none of the six compounds with skin reactions in man had related problems in animal studies, as this type of idiosyncratic reaction is difficult to detect in animals. However, six of the seven compounds with cardiovascular reactions in man had related findings in the animal studies (Table 7.3).

Time-scale for animals and man

The relationship of duration of dosing in animals to the duration in man must also be considered. For example, can a period of three months in a study with laboratory animals be compared with the same time period for humans? As shown in Table 7.4, the life span is approximately 30 months for the rat, 150 months for the dog and

Table 7.4 Relationship between life span, heart and respiration rate for animals and man

	Rat	*Dog*	*Human*
Life span (month)	30	150	900
Heart rate / minute	350	100	70
Respiration rate / minute	100	25	20

900 months for humans. It may be more appropriate to consider time-scales in relation to physiological parameters such as the heart and respiration rate. On this basis, one could propose that 12 months exposure of a drug to humans is comparable to three to six months in the dog and one to three months in the rat.

A proposal

The duration of toxicity studies to support repeated dosing in humans should be discussed on a more scientific basis. Animal data are essential for the safety assessment of new drugs, particularly when initiating clinical trials where little or no human data are available. However, as discussed above, three months of exposure to a test drug in animals may be comparable to much longer than six months exposure in man. Also, most of the toxic effects (excluding cancer) produced in repeated dose studies in animals are identified by 3-month studies. It is therefore proposed that four weeks repeated dosing in animals is sufficient to support studies in humans up to four weeks. Following this, three months repeated dose toxicity studies should be recommended as the minimum duration to support repeated dosing of longer than four weeks in all phases of clinical investigation. Long-term dosing in humans, such as that over six months, can only be supported by human data which are accumulated by the step-wise process of clinical investigation.

References

Contrera JF, Aub D, Barbehenn E *et al.* (1993). A retrospective comparison of the results of six and twelve month non-rodent toxicity studies. *Adverse Drug Reactions and Toxicological Reviews*, **12**(1), 63–76.

Igarashi T (1992). Is the 12-month treatment essential for the repeated dose study? In D'Arcy PF and Harron DWG (eds.) *Proceedings of the First International Conference on Harmonisation, Brussels, 1991*. Belfast: Queens University Press. pp. 248–250.

Igarashi T (1993). A review of the Japanese Pharmaceutical Manufacturers' Association database currently established to examine retrospectively the value of long-term animal toxicology studies. *Adverse Drug Reactions and Toxicological Reviews*, **12**(1), 35–52

JPMA (1993). Nonclinical Evaluation Committee Report, JPMA Documentation No. 61 (in Japanese)

JPMA (1994). Nonclinical Evaluation Committee Report, JPMA Documentation No. 65 (in Japanese)

Lumley CE, Parkinson C and Walker SR (1993). The value of the dog in long-term toxicity studies. The CMR International Toxicology Database. *Adverse Drug Reactions and Toxicological Reviews*, **12**(1), 53–61

8 The duration of toxicity studies required to support repeated dosing in clinical investigation – a clinician's opinion

JOHN ALEXANDER

Summary

1. The rodent carcinogenicity study is frequently the key rate-limiting step for development of many compounds for chronic therapy. Because of the long duration, cost and chemical requirements of these studies, it is worth reconsidering their importance.
2. About one-half of all chemicals (whether natural or synthetic) tested at the maximum tolerated dose are rodent carcinogens. However, evidence is inconclusive or inconsistent regarding their increased risk of cancer in man. It is therefore urgent to study the results of company and regulatory experiences of the sensitivity and specificity of the rodent bioassay.
3. It is proposed that the rodent carcinogenicity study should not be required for marketing approval unless there is a suspicious chemical structure, evidence of mutagenicity or toxicity findings of concern. The rodent carcinogenicity tests should, however, be initiated before the new drug application is submitted for all drugs, with some exceptions, such as drugs for cancer and AIDS.

Healthcare reform, harmonisation discussions and AIDS, together with business redesign currently underway in many pharmaceutical companies, have created a climate of change and an examination of the fundamentals of all of the activities in research and especially in drug development.

Healthcare reform, with mandatory reductions in government reimbursements and greater price sensitivity in every country, has forced pharmaceutical companies to examine carefully all of their practices to find ways that costs can be reduced. In the USA this process is called reengineering and a book called, *Reengineering the Corporation: A Manifesto for Business Revolution* (Hammer and Champy, 1993) has been on the best seller list for many months, reflecting the intense effort that is underway to control costs and improve business processes and performance in the USA. In the pharmaceutical industry, one area of focus of these reengineering and redesign efforts has been to find ways of speeding drug development and approval. Time rather than money has been the main emphasis. As an example, Figure 8.1 shows sales revenue for a major

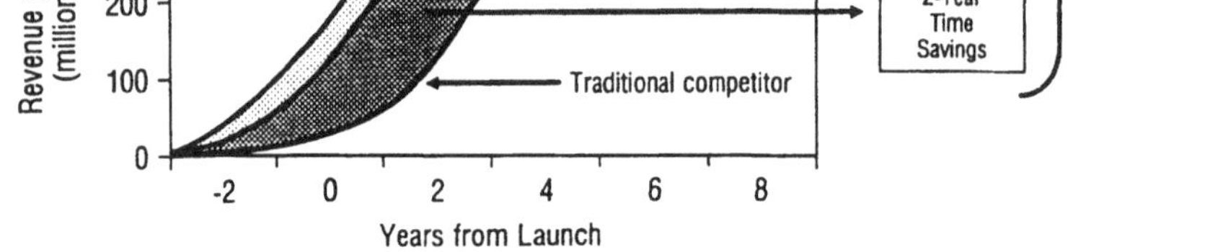

Figure 8.1 Sales revenue implications of reducing development time by two years for a major drug. Two benefits can be reaped: the drug is earning patent-protected revenues for an additional two years (dark tint), and the drug reaches greater overall peak revenues by virtue of earlier market positioning (light tint). Reproduced by permission of Boston Consulting Group.
*Time-based competitors can at a minimum reap additional patent-protected revenues (middle curve) or higher overall revenues due to preferential market positioning (upper curve). This translates into $400–600 million in additional net present value for each major drug.

drug which peaks at about $500 million. The traditional competitor comes later to the market and never really achieves this level of sales. The difference in sales between these competitors, resulting from a two-year difference in bringing a similar drug to market, is about $400–600 million. In other words, each day of delay for an important drug with sales of $300 million at the time of patent expiry costs $1 million.

Expedited approval

In the past, the Food and Drug Administration (FDA) data requirements have dictated developmental strategy. While this was always under some debate, the need to rapidly develop drugs for AIDS created tremendous pressures for change. In order to speed the approval of new drugs for AIDS in the USA, it has been possible to obtain conditional approval after only Phase II clinical testing with requirements to complete Phase III investigations. When faced with a universally fatal illness, it seems very appropriate to allow rapid approval before complete clinical and toxicological data are available. The benefits of early approval clearly outweigh the risks. A similar situation exists for cancer chemotherapy where relatively few patients are needed for approval and historical controls are frequently adequate. In addition, carcinogenicity testing is not usually required.

Critical path analysis

We need to extend this thinking to other drugs that may not be life saving. One area that requires urgent discussion is the animal carcinogenicity studies that are required for most drugs intended for chronic therapy. In project planning it has been popular to use critical path analysis as a way of identifying areas where time can be saved. What has not been fully appreciated is that the rodent carcinogenicity study is frequently the key rate-limiting step for development of many compounds for chronic therapy (Figure 8.2). About three years are required to conduct and report the results of the carcinogenicity study; therefore no drug can be developed in less than three years. To prevent delays the carcinogenicity study needs to be initiated very early in the development process, with range-finding toxicological

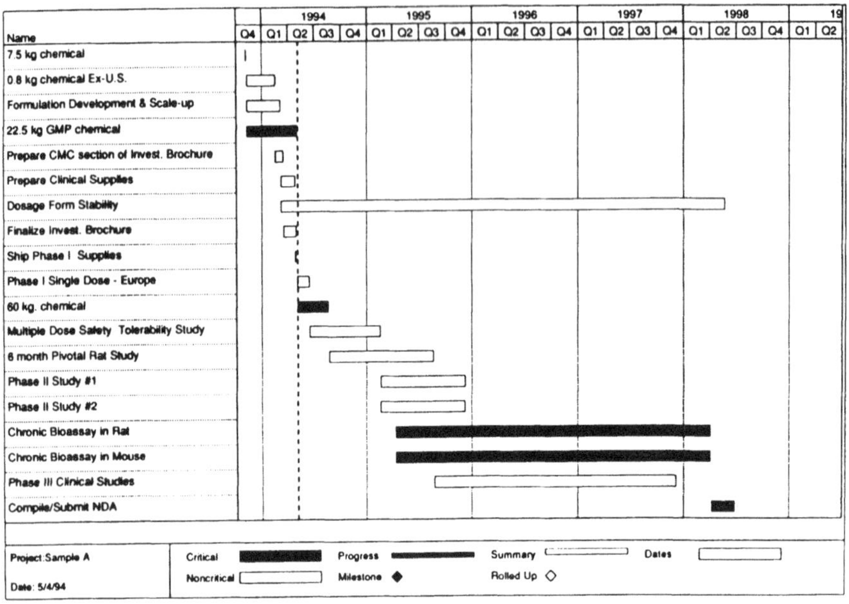

Figure 8.2 Critical path analysis for a compound in development

studies to find the maximum tolerated dose (MTD), and before much of the key clinical data is available to determine the true value of the drug. Because of the long duration, cost and chemical requirements of these carcinogenicity studies, it is worth reconsidering their importance. This will be the focus of my proposal.

Carcinogenicity studies

Recent information about cancer epidemiology and prevention (Table 8.1) indicates that about 80% of the cancer cases in the USA may be caused by environmental factors including drugs. It is very difficult to find conclusive evidence for a carcinogen because of the long time interval between the exposure and the diagnosis of cancer, and most carcinogens cause cancer in only a small proportion of those exposed and increase risk only modestly. It is also now being recognised that diet is probably of great importance in the development of cancer. At this time it has been established that there are

Table 8.1 Cancer epidemiology and prevention

- 80% of cancer cases in the USA may be caused by environmental factors
- Conclusive evidence is difficult due to the long time between exposure and diagnosis
- Most carcinogens cause cancer in only a small portion of those exposed
- Diet is of great importance
- Most cancers are caused by agents that increase risk only modestly
- About 20 chemicals are known to be carcinogenic in humans
- Many compounds can induce cancer in animals, but evidence is inconclusive or inconsistent regarding increased risk in man

Adapted from Li and Gann (1994)

about 20 chemicals that are known to be carcinogenic in man including well-known agents such as tobacco and smoking.

A recent review (Li and Gann, 1994) points out that only 20 chemicals, out of a universe of 60,000 chemicals in daily use, are known to be carcinogenic in humans (Table 8.2). Drugs that are clearly recognised as carcinogens include alkylating agents, androgenic steroids, synthetic oestrogens, phenacetin and immunosuppressive drugs. Ames and Gold (1990) pointed out that about half of all chemicals (whether natural or synthetic) tested at the MTD are rodent carcinogens. However, evidence is inconclusive or inconsistent regarding their increased risk of cancer in man (Li and Gann, 1994). This is the framework in which we must consider the rodent carcinogenicity study.

Ideally, it is necessary to present the sensitivity, specificity and predictive value of the rodent carcinogenicity test as would be done with any other diagnostic test (Figure 8.3). This is the type of data that establishes the validity of a screening test. Looking objectively at the rodent cancer bioassay, it must be recognised that it is a screening test, but the confirmatory test is epidemiology in man. It is known that there are clear false negatives such as nicotine and alcohol, and a very significant number of false positives. However, it is important that more data is collected from company and regulatory agency records in order to improve the definition of the test, by answering the questions posed in Table 8.3.

Table 8.2 Established environmental causes of human cancer

Carcinogen	*Cancer site or associate neoplasm*
Alcoholic beverages	Liver, oesophagus, mouth, pharynx, larynx
Alkylating agents (melphalan, cyclophosphamide, chlorambucil, nitrosoureas), epipodophyllotoxins	Acute myelocytic leukemia, bladder (cyclophosphamide)
Androgenic steroids	Liver
Aromatic amines	Bladder
Arsenic (inorganic)	Lung, skin
Asbestos	Lung, pleura, peritoneum, pericardium
Benzene	Acute myeloctyic leukemia
bis-Chloromethyl ether	Lung
Chromium	Lung
Chronic hepatitis B infection	Liver
Diethylstilbestrol (pre-natal exposure)	Vagina (adenocarcinoma)
Epstein–Barr virus	Nasopharyngeal Burkitt's lymphoma
HTLV-I	Adult T cell leukemia/lymphoma
Immunosuppressive drugs (azathioprine, cyclosporine)	Non-Hodgkin's lymphoma
Ionising radiation	Almost all organs
Isopropyl alcohol production	Nasal sinuses
Mustard gas	Lung, larynx, nasal sinuses
Nickel dust	Lung, nasal sinuses
Phenacetin	Renal pelvis, bladder
Polycyclic hydrocarbons	Lung, scrotum, skin (sqamous carcinoma)
Sunlight (UV)	Skin, intraocular melanoma
Schistosomiasis	Bladder
Synthetic oestrogens	Endometrium
Tobacco	Lung, mouth, pharynx, larynx, oesophagus, pancreas, bladder, kidney, renal pelvis
Vinyl chloride	Liver (angiosarcoma)
Wood dust	Nasal sinuses

Adapted from Li and Gann (1994)

	Cancer in man	
Carcinogenic in animals	Present	Absent
Positive	TP	FP
Negative	FN	TN

$$\text{Sensitivity} = \frac{\text{TP}}{\text{TP} + \text{FN}}$$

$$\text{Specificity} = \frac{\text{TN}}{\text{TP} + \text{FP}}$$

$$\text{Specificity} = \frac{\text{TP}}{\text{TP} + \text{FP}}$$

Figure 8.3 Rodent carcinogenicity bioassay

Proposal

As a general principle we should rely to a greater degree on the clinical judgements of risk and benefit as we plan our drug development programmes and the clinical and toxicological studies. It has been generally established that carcinogenicity testing for life threatening diseases can be completed after approval or even not conducted at all.

My proposal is that while we debate the value of the rodent carcinogenicity study, it should not be the rate-limiting step for drug development and should not be required for approval unless there is a suspicious chemical structure, evidence of mutagenicity or toxicity findings of concern (Table 8.4). The rodent carcinogenicity tests should be initiated before the new drug application is submitted for all drugs, again with some exceptions for drugs for cancer, AIDS, etc. Finally, it is urgent to study and present the results of company and regulatory experiences of the sensitivity and specificity of rodent bioassay. The only way to truly determine increased cancer risk of drugs is careful epidemiological studies in man. We

Table 8.3 Questions related to animal carcinogenicity studies

- What is the scientific basis of these studies? We use large doses of drugs over the lifetime of a small number of animals rather than the clinical experience which will usually be a much smaller dose over a shorter duration of time. Is this rational?
- How many drugs that have been introduced into medicine before the current required carcinogenicity studies have been shown to cause cancer or increase the risk?
- How many drugs have been dropped from development because of tumours found in animal studies? Are these true or false positives?
- What has been the clinical experience with drugs that have shown evidence of carcinogenicity in animal studies? Would the epidemiological data be good enough for us to even know?
- Can analysis of chemical structures, mutagenicity studies, human liver cell metabolic studies and new cell line models with known carcinogens provide enough evidence for or against conducting a chronic animal study?
- If the animal carcinogenicity studies cannot be eliminated, can they be improved? Can they be shortened? What animals should be tested to gain the most information? Do we really need the MTD?

also need to find better ways in which drug epidemiological data would be available to assess cancer risk.

Regarding other toxicological studies, again we need to be guided by risk/benefit considerations. It is reasonable to test drugs in animals before initiation of studies in man, but it is important to consider what the toxicological studies contribute once a new drug is in clinical development. Once a drug is in man, we are guided most by the human experience we have obtained. While the findings in animal studies may guide us to look for certain adverse findings in man, most of these tests would be done in any case. The animal studies can help with the causality assessment, but are they worth the cost in terms of false positive findings and critical resources of limited drug supplies? While I may accept the idea that we must do everything possible in animals to identify toxicity for drugs that may be used as preventive agents in healthy people, such as those with cardiovascular risk factors, I am not sure they are needed for many potentially very beneficial agents.

Table 8.4 Proposal

GENERAL:

- Greater reliance of risk/benefit considerations from medical perspective

RODENT CARCINOGENICITY BIOASSAY:

- Not a requirement for approval when:
  - Life threatening disease
  - When the following exist:
    1. Not a suspicious chemical structure
    2. Negative mutagenicity tests
    3. Absence of suggestive changes in short-term toxicity tests
- Should be initiated before new drug application
- Additional studies are needed to justify routine use

As clinicians are involved in these considerations, we are faced with regulations rather than data that justify the animal studies. I look forward to an examination of the data that guides our selection of animal toxicity studies, and believe that these discussions will be a tremendous opportunity for rational drug development.

References

Ames BN and Gold LS (1990). Chemical carcinogenesis: too many rodent carcinogens. *Proc Natl Acad Sci*, **87**, 7772–7776

Hammer M and Champy J (1993). *Reengineering the Corporation: A Manifesto for Business Revolution*. Prentice Hall, New York

Li, F and Gann, P (1994). Cancer epidemiology and prevention. In: Ruberenstein, R (ed.) *Scientific American Medicine Inc*, New York, 12:I:2–9

9 Reproductive and developmental toxicity studies required to support the inclusion of women and children in clinical trials – a toxicologist's opinion

KURT SUTER

Summary

1. The ICH harmonised tripartite guideline on the detection of toxicity to reproduction for medicinal products can be regarded as a major breakthrough which will lead to studies of improved scientific quality, less duplication of work, fewer animals being used and, hopefully, will speed up drug development. However, it does not specify how the proposed designs and strategies are to be brought into line with the clinical development process and does not indicate the minimum requirements for the inclusion of women of childbearing potential in clinical trials.

2. It is proposed that the minimum set of reproductive toxicity studies performed to permit the inclusion of women should contain an assessment of embryo/foetal development, including morphological assessment of the foetuses, as well as an assessment of fertility and early embryonic development. For the inclusion of males, histopathological assessments of testis and epididymus tissues from repeated dose toxicity studies are necessary.

3. Many medicines are regularly prescribed to children and for certain indications it is already clear at the beginning of development that children will be part of the patient population. At least in these instances preclinical safety testing in the juvenile organism should be made part of the development process. Within the framework of the ICH guideline, there are several options for the testing of juvenile animals.

Introduction

Decisions on the extent of preclinical testing necessary before women of childbearing age and children can be included in clinical trials are complex. Several factors, among them the clinical/biological risk situation, guideline requirements, pharmacological and kinetic properties of the drug under investigation as well as certain needs of the drug development process, must be taken into consideration. This paper will concentrate on the more general aspects of the clinical/biological risk situation as well as on the issue of a guideline. The latter is of particular interest because, as a result of the second meeting of the International Conference on Harmonisation of Technical Requirements for the Registration of Pharmaceuticals for Human Use (ICH2), held in Orlando in October 1993, a guideline on the "Detection of Toxicity to Reproduction for Medicinal Products" has been issued (EC Commission, 1993) which can be expected to be adopted soon by the regulatory bodies of the European Union, Japan and the USA. Testing requirements should always be seen within the practical context of drug development. Therefore some proposals on how certain study types could be scheduled within the development process are also made. Since the regulatory situation thus far is not clear, the proposals have to be seen as a basis for discussions rather than as solutions of a problem.

ICH harmonised tripartite guideline on the detection of toxicity to reproduction for medicinal products

The ICH guideline can be regarded as a major breakthrough which will lead to studies of improved scientific quality, less duplication of work, fewer animals being used and, hopefully, will speed up drug development. Discussions now being conducted on the preclinical requirements for the inclusion of women of childbearing age and children into clinical trials should be based on this new guideline. Most of the experimental procedures and designs recommended by this ICH guideline are by no means revolutionary. In fact, most of them are already contained in one way or another in the classical Segment I, II and III approaches presently in effect, e.g. in the USA and Japan. The most important achievement of the guideline is the fact that the selection of the study designs is left to the scientific judgement of the investigator as long as certain basic rules are followed. It is evident that this flexibility is the best prerequisite to achieve the aim of reproduction toxicity testing, which is to reveal any adverse effect of one or more active substance(s) on mammalian reproduction.

The guideline is based on the principle that in one species (usually the rat) reproductive toxicity testing has to cover a full reproduction cycle, i.e. treatment should last from conception to sexual maturity. This can be done either with one study or with several studies in which animals are treated during defined stages of reproduction. There should be a minimum overlap of one day between the different studies. Although the guideline gives some recommendations, it is up to the investigator to choose the appropriate combination of studies. The rationale for the selection, however, has to be provided.

Some other guiding principles are as follows:

- The best possible use should be made of any existing additional toxicological, pharmacological and kinetic information. Repeated dose toxicity studies can provide important information regarding potential effects on reproduction, particularly on male fertility. The premating period for male rats may be reduced to four weeks (saving six weeks if compared with the old guideline) if sufficient information on potential effects on spermatogenesis is provided by means of a careful histopathological investigation performed in repeated dose toxicity studies.
- Tests on physical development, sensory functions and behaviour are to be included, even though the guideline states that it is not possible to recommend specific tests.
- Morphological changes are to be assessed in two different species (usually the rat and rabbit).
- A minimal number of animals should be used, and suffering should be avoided.

The high degree of freedom granted to the investigator is remarkable. It is not totally surprising that in the same guideline a remark of caution is also made: *"It is anticipated that, initially, preference will be given (by the investigator) to designs that do not differ too radically from those of established guidelines for medicinal products"*. A proposal for a

Table 9.1 ICH guideline: "the most probable option"

Study 1	*Study 2*	*Study 3*
Fertility and early embryonic development (study treatment period according to the Japanese guidelines; dissection, however, in mid pregnancy)	Pre- and post-natal development including maternal function (new type of study – treatment from implantation to weaning, assessment of physical and functional development)	Embryo/foetal development (study according to the Food and Drug Administration (FDA) guidelines, dissection shortly before term)

"moderate" new design is given under the term "the most probable option". It consists of three studies as shown in Table 9.1.

In addition to the "most probable option" which, according to the number of rodent studies performed, is a three-study design, suggestions are given in the guideline for a one-study design and various two-study designs, thus underlining and demonstrating flexibility. It is to be hoped that the spirit of the ICH guideline in its full extent will become part of the national guidelines.

Inclusion of women (and men) in clinical trials

In spite of its positive aspects, the ICH guideline also has some serious drawbacks. It fails to specify how the proposed designs and strategies are to be brought into line with the clinical development process. Are all three studies, e.g. those of the "most probable option", necessary to permit the inclusion of women of childbearing potential into clinical trials, or is it acceptable to perform the studies in a sequential order during the drug development process? If this is the case, what are the minimum requirements for the inclusion of women? Similar considerations have to be made for male volunteers/patients of reproductive age. Even before the ICH guideline was written, this was an area not without controversy, as demonstrated by differing requirements in different countries.

In Europe and the USA no mammalian reproduction tests are required for the first clinical trials in male volunteers. For the inclusion of women of childbearing age in clinical Phase I studies,

Segment II animal studies are required in Europe, and in the USA, in addition, a Segment I study has to be performed. In Japan a fertility study in male animals is needed for the inclusion of men into clinical trials, and a full set of reproduction studies (Segment I, II and III) is required for the initiation of clinical Phase I studies in women.

At present the issue of animal tests required for the inclusion of volunteers/patients into clinical trials is further complicated by suggestions that women should become part of such trials as early as possible. In the past there seemed to be a general consensus that, as far as possible, only male volunteers/patients should be included in first clinical trials. This mainly stemmed from the assumption that the risk which is associated with the inadvertent exposure of embryos in an undiagnosed early pregnancy is not acceptable. It is now being pointed out, particularly in the USA, that the early enrolment of women in clinical trials might not only be of benefit in regard to safety, but is actually a necessity. It is evident that, from the ethical as well as scientific points of view, differences in basic requirements for safety assessment between countries as well as genders are not justified. Therefore, in addition to the harmonisation of the preclinical study designs, standards in relation to minimal requirements and timing of toxicological safety assessment in conjunction with the clinical testing phases are urgently needed.

The study designs as proposed in the ICH guideline were developed with registration in mind. If performed to their full extent, studies would be sufficient for the inclusion of male and female volunteers into clinical trials, assuming that no reproduction problem has been identified. For the drug development process the question of whether a full set of animal tests is necessary before any male or female volunteer/patient can be included in an early clinical trial is of high practical importance.

A guiding principle for defining requirements for animal tests relates to clinical risk. Among other factors, the potential endpoints affected during treatment are of special importance (Table 9.2). For clinical trials in males these endpoints are altered sexual behaviour and fertility effects. For women in clinical trials, additional potential endpoints are early gestation, embryonal death, structural abnormalities, altered embryonal growth and delayed functional effects in the offspring. For toxicological testing preceding clinical trials these endpoints are of primary interest. On the other hand, late

Table 9.2 Main reproductive/developmental risks of volunteers in Phase I clinical trials

	Male volunteers	*Female volunteers*
Reproductive toxicity risk		
alteration in sexual behaviour	X	X
onset of puberty		
effects on menstrual cycle		X
fertility	X	X
gestation		X
parturition		
lactation		
Developmental toxicity risk (effects in progeny)		
death		X
structural abnormality		X
altered growth		X
functional deficits		X

gestation/parturition and lactation are conditions usually excluded from clinical trials. Consequently these endpoints may be postponed and assessed at a later stage of development.

Another important question is whether, for initial, small-scale clinical trials being conducted under strictly controlled conditions, all identified potential endpoints should be included in the animal tests on a mandatory basis. In this context, testing for delayed functional and behavioural effects in the offspring as well as testing for male fertility effects are of interest. Since there are, as of yet, no recognised and approved methods available for the testing of functional and behavioural deficits, these tests should not be made a mandatory part of *early* testing for teratogenic effects. In respect to male fertility effects, experience has demonstrated that histopathological investigation of testicular and epididymal tissues from repeated dose studies leads to a reliable identification of compounds interfering with the process of spermatogenesis. These investigations reduce the potential risk to an acceptable level, and should be sufficient to permit the inclusion of males into small-scale first clinical trials.

From these considerations, it follows that the minimum set of reproductive toxicity studies performed to permit the inclusion of women should contain an assessment of embryo/foetal development, including morphological assessment of the foetuses, as well as an assessment of fertility and early embryonic development (Table 9.3). For the inclusion of males, histopathological assessments of testis and epididymis tissues from repeated dose toxicity studies are necessary. Since, in the usual toxicological testing sequence, histopathological information on the testis and epididymis is available earlier than information on fertility and embryonal/foetal development, it is still likely that first clinical trials will be performed with male volunteers/patients in the future. Initiation of the appropriate animal studies immediately after transition into Phase I will allow the inclusion of female volunteers into clinical trials during the second half of Phase I.

If a full set of reproductive toxicity studies is not performed during Phase I of clinical testing, information on the aspects not tested should be provided in clinical Phases II and III, when more patients are included into trials (Table 9.3).

Table 9.3 Preclinical information required for inclusion of male and female volunteers/patients into clinical trials

	Male healthy volunteers/ patients	*Women of childbearing potential*
Phase I	Testes weight in 4-week toxicity studies (rats and dogs). Histopathological assessment of testes and epididymides in 4-week toxicity studies.	Fertility and early embryonic development. Embryo/foetal development – morphological effects (two species).
Phase II	Fertility (e.g. within the frame of fertility and early embryonic development).	No additional tests.
Phase III	No additional tests.	Study of pre- and post-natal development including functional and behavioural development.

Inclusion of children in clinical trials

It is interesting to note that, although it is stated in the ICH guideline that testing for reproduction effects should cover a full reproduction cycle, the proposed study designs and strategies do not make suggestions for the period starting from weaning until attainment of sexual maturity. Already the classical Segment I, II and III approach was developed under the assumption that drugs are primarily developed for adults, thus making preclinical safety testing in the juvenile organism not mandatory. Paediatric indications are usually entered on a case by case basis after the market approval for an adult indication has been granted. Obviously there is a considerable number of drugs regularly prescribed to children, and for certain drugs it is already clear at the beginning of development that they will ultimately also be prescribed to children, for example, drugs in the indications asthma and epilepsy. At least in these instances preclinical safety testing in the juvenile organism should be made part of the development process.

The only standard study design fully covering the juvenile period is the two-generation study as designed for the testing of agrochemical products or food additives. Since, from a practical point of view, this study design will hardly be applied to pharmaceutical products, some additional thoughts are necessary on how toxicological testing in juvenile animals can be done within the concept of the ICH guideline.

The species of choice for such studies is the rat, providing that it had been found adequate for repeated dose and reproductive toxicity studies as well as being relevant for the human situation. Using the same species for preclinical testing assures that the results obtained can be related and interpreted, making it unnecessary to use a second species.

Potential endpoints relevant for the risk situation in children and adolescents are shown in Table 9.4. They include alterations to sexual behaviour, onset of puberty, oestrus cycle, fertility, growth and function. These endpoints could be tested in animal studies using the same techniques as employed for other reproduction studies. However, in addition to the usual reproduction and developmental endpoints, other endpoints should also be considered because of the special conditions found in a developing animal, including receptor sensitivity, drug disposition and kinetics, the haematological system and the immunological system. Investigations similar to those in a

Table 9.4 Main reproductive/developmental risks of children and adolescents exposed to pharmaceutical products

	Male children	*Female children*
Reproductive toxicity risk		
sexual behaviour	X	X
onset of puberty	X	X
effects on menstrual cycle		X
fertility	X	X
gestation		
parturition		
lactation		
Developmental toxicity risk		
death		
structural abnormality		
altered growth	X	X
functional deficits	X	X
toxicity		
General toxicity		

prolonged toxicity study should be included, e.g. haematological, clinical chemistry and histopathological assessments.

Because of the small size of juvenile animals, invasive techniques can in most instances only be applied toward the end of the study, i.e. when sexual maturity has been reached. Fertility and sexual behaviour should not be assessed if these aspects have already been dealt with in a fertility and early embryonic development study.

Within the framework of the ICH guideline the following options for the testing of juvenile animals can be foreseen: (i) prolonging the pre- and post-natal study or a similar study and extending the treatment period beyond weaning (by 8–10 weeks) until the attainment of sexual maturity; and (ii) setting up a special study covering the period between the end of weaning and attainment of sexual maturity.

The technical details of a study in juvenile animals should be determined by the clinical situation in which the drug is to be used.

References

Commission of the European Communities (1993). Committee for Proprietary Medicinal Products, Note for Guidance. Detection of toxicity to reproduction for medicinal products (III/3387/93 FINAL).

SECTION III

Proposals and the Way Forward

Proposals and the way forward

Finding the right strategy with regard to the timing of toxicological studies conducted to support clinical trials should enable the seamless development of new medicines for therapeutic use. One of the objectives of this CMR meeting was to bring together experienced pharmaceutical toxicologists and clinicians from around the world to discuss the toxicity studies they believed were justified to support the various stages of clinical development. Three of the main considerations in any developmental strategy were identified for deliberation, and some general questions were posed in order to focus the discussions (Table 1). The participants were split into equal sized groups consisting of toxicologists and clinicians with the remit to reach a consensus on a scientifically and ethically justifiable approach to toxicity testing for their particular topic.

Each discussion group had just under three hours in which to formulate a consensus proposal on its allocated topic. Due to the short time available, it was not possible to discuss all situations or types of compounds. The proposals therefore relate to compounds generally for oral administration and intended to treat non-life-threatening conditions. It was, however, not possible to reach a consensus on every issue, and in these situations the majority view was proposed. The proposals were then presented by the groups' rapporteurs to the whole meeting along with how the groups had arrived at their recommendations. These proposals have been reproduced in the following chapters, together with lists of the members of each group.

There was considerable discussion on each topic and some of the areas of disagreement have been highlighted. Although a consensus was not reached on every issue, it is hoped that these proposals will contribute to the wider discussions currently taking place on this topic. They provide a starting point from which to develop an international consensus on the appropriate timing of toxicity studies in relation to clinical trials.

Table 1 Discussion group topics

1. Initiating Phase I clinical trials: what is the minimum non-clinical package necessary?
   - *What general toxicology is needed before single-dose studies in volunteers?*
   - *How much genetic toxicology?*
   - *What about* in vitro *screens? How much toxicokinetics and metabolism data?*
   - *Does one have to do fertility studies before Phase I?*
   - *Is there justification for the Japanese requirement for an antigenicity study?*

2. Duration of studies required to support repeat-dosing in man in all phases of clinical trials.
   - *The merits of the FDA guidelines compared to those of the EU and Japan.*
   - *The requirement for carcinogenicity studies for long-term trials.*
   - *What would be an ideal approach?*
   - *How is it best (or quickest) to report these animal studies?*
   - *Are regulatory guidelines counter-productive?*

3. Timing of reproductive and developmental studies in relation to clinical trials.
   - *The consequences of the new ICH guideline.*
   - *The implication of early recruitment of female volunteers into clinical studies.*
   - *Problems with reproductive toxicology studies becoming an earlier component of the safety assessment programme.*
   - *Are there adequate alternative studies? Studies necessary to allow clinical trials in children.*

10 The minimum non-clinical package for initiating Phase I clinical trials

MICHAEL JACKSON and JACK DEAN

Introduction

First exposure of humans to a new candidate medicine is a major step in both ethical and development terms. Development speed and flexibility are particularly critical, since the early preclinical evaluation and initial assessment in the clinic will determine the abandonment or progression of a compound before extensive resources have been employed. There is therefore a compelling case to design any preclinical package to allow the first exposure to man to be primarily consistent with the provision of an adequate safety evaluation, while being economic of resources.

There is a powerful argument for allowing the pharmaceutical industry to progress to Phase I studies in healthy volunteers without any regulatory approval, in order to encourage speed and flexibility. Such an opportunity exists in certain European territories where Ethics Review Boards approve Phase I studies in healthy volunteers. Experience of this system has shown that such a process contains rigorous safety checks with frequent and close interactions between the various disciplines involved. In those territories where studies in healthy volunteers require national regulatory approval there is a strong view from the pharmaceutical industry that regulatory agencies should review their processes so as to allow, as far as possible, maximum flexibility at this stage of drug development.

Phase I clinical studies – terms of reference

The usual practice is for multiple-dose administration in man to be preceded by a single-dose study in male volunteers. Within clinical pharmacology practice, the term single-dose is taken to encompass up to three doses with an adequate wash-out period between each dose (generally at least one week) depending on the pharmacokinetics of the compound.

The proposed preclinical package is designed to support administration to healthy adult males; restricting the subject population to males avoids extensive, and potentially delaying, reproductive toxicology. This toxicology package is considered sufficient to allow radio-labelled studies if local regulations concerning administration of radio-labelled materials are met. Products derived from biotechnology, however, would not necessarily be embraced appropriately by this proposed approach and deserve case by case consideration.

The flexible approach

Flexibility of approach allows a preclinical package that is geared to the objectives of Phase I studies. Pragmatism tends to bias approaches in exploratory development towards either *investigational* or *development* categories, which are defined in Table 10.1. In practice, a spectrum of approaches applies so that a 'mix-and-match' is formulated in accordance with objectives sought in the human studies.

Adoption of the *development* model implies that a candidate medicine has been selected for which there is an optimistic outlook that progress towards full development will be straight forward. By contrast, the *investigational* model is likely to be used for compounds that require some critical preliminary questions to be answered before being selected for development. Given the uncertainty of the investigational process, it is sensible to use resources economically. On the other hand, regulatory robustness is appropriate for the *development* model so that additional time is not wasted by having to repeat studies.

Implications for preclinical package

For full advantage to be gained from the flexible approach outlined above, the extent of preclinical work should be geared to the objectives of the early clinical studies. However, provision of appropriate safety data remains paramount. Common to both *investigational* and *development* models are adequate delineation of the test article quality from

Table 10.1 Review of criteria that apply to investigational vs development approaches

Criterion	*Investigational*	*Development*	*Approaches/comments*
Novelty	++	+	The *investigational* approach is more likely to be appropriate for compounds for which previous experience with a drug class is absent and responses in animals/man may be difficult to predict.
Objective	Selection process	Safety/ tolerance dose setting/ efficacy	The *investigational* model will often apply to compounds for which there is no firm commitment to development prior to appropriate characterisation. This contrasts with adoption of a *development* model, where previous experience with the drug class or application of the *investigational* approach has led to sufficient development intent and application of resources.
Compound candidates	>1	1	By implication the candidate selection process is determined by the availability of alternative compounds that may have to be screened so as to avoid unacceptable risk that might emerge from the toxicology/clinical pharmacology studies on the initial compound.
Dose range in Phase I clinical studies	Single (one dose only)	'Single' (up to three doses)	In the *development* strategy the acute 3-dose concept must allow adequate wash-out periods between exposures.
Phase I dose levels	May be sub-therapeutic	'Stretching'	In an *investigational* approach a critical question (i.e., bioavailability) may be answerable by administration of a very low dose. This has implications for dose levels utilised in the preclinical programme and compound supply. In contrast the *development* model will seek to establish maximum tolerability levels in humans.

Table 10.1 (continued)

Criterion	*Investigational*	*Development*	*Approaches/comments*
Phase I endpoints	PK or PK/PD focus	PK/PD broad	Here the *investigational* model may focus simply on pharmacokinetic (PK) evaluation whereas in *development* information on tolerability will demand pharmacodynamic (PD) assessment as well as provision of PK data.
Phase I subject population size	Small	Larger	For the *investigational* approach the nature of the question posed may allow the study population size to be comparatively small. In *development* there is a need for regulatory robustness as these will be pivotal studies for registration purposes.
Outcome	Move compound to development mode or if inappropriate return to alternative investigational compounds	Move to full development or abandon and possibly adopt *investigational* approach	View as interactive cycles between *investigational* and *development* mode.
Extent of preclinical safety investigation	Minimal – sufficient to permit a focussed question to be answered	Appropriate to allow smooth progression towards clinical trials	In the *development* mode the assumption is success so that the animal work must satisfy accepted regulatory needs. Thus this work must always be conducted to full GLP.

pharmacy/Chemistry Manufacturing Controls (CMC) and appropriate toxicokinetics by which safety can be monitored on the basis of systemic exposure.

Within the battery of current preclinical test procedures, there is little scope for differences in genetic toxicology and safety pharmacology between the two models. There is, however, the possibility of greater flexibility in the design of the general toxicology package.

Table 10.2 itemises the toxicology packages appropriate for each model, which are commented on below.

Genetic toxicology

A testing programme should allow for detection of both point mutations and clastogenicity. This is usually done by suitable *in vitro* bacterial tests and an *in vivo* micronucleus test. Any further work to satisfy registration requirements can be left to a later stage. A positive test in the bacterial screen would not necessarily dictate abandonment of the compound. There is general agreement that further *in vivo* tests or mechanistic approaches may allow such a result to be rationalised in terms of safety for human volunteers. A clear positive in an *in vivo* clastogenicity test would normally preclude progression to healthy subjects.

Safety pharmacology

This element of preclinical safety is seen to be particularly apposite to the first exposure of humans to a candidate medicine. The dose levels employed usually correspond to those likely to be attained in humans. Pharmacodynamic responses are examined in far more detail than in toxicity tests. The key battery comprises evaluation of those systems (cardiovascular/CNS/respiratory) that are generally most responsive to acute exposure, and in this sense are particularly vital to the well-being of the human subject. Safety pharmacology exploring, for example, the renal and/or gastro-intestinal systems may need to be considered if the pharmacology in animals or class relationships suggest the possibility of adverse effects. It is important to select appropriately sensitive species for this area of work. This may on occasion be the species/strain used in the research discovery phase. There may also be a reason for employing toxicokinetics in safety pharmacology studies,

Table 10.2 Toxicology to support human studies – early Phase I

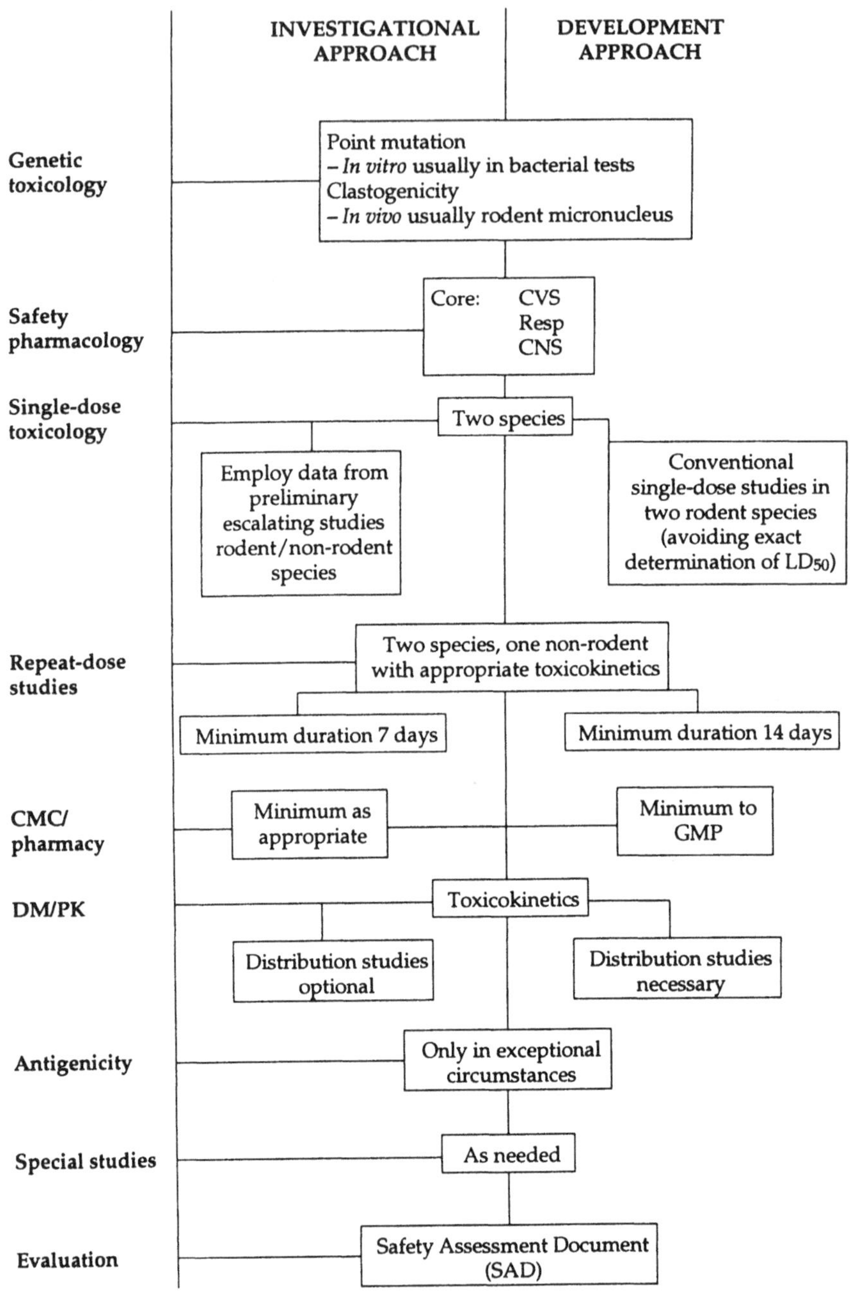

although this may be unnecessary if the compound is administered intravenously.

General toxicity

In this area the intention is to identify, as far as possible, target organs/systems and establish safety margins on the basis of systemic exposure. For both *investigational* and *development* approaches, a reasonable idea of the safety margin following single dosing is needed. This may be gleaned from preliminary incremental dosing prior to repeat-dose studies. For *investigational* approaches, initial dose-escalating studies in rodents and non-rodents give valuable high dosage information which can also be used in selecting doses for the repeat-dose studies. Conventional single-dose toxicology in two rodent species can therefore be reserved for the *development* model in order to satisfy regulatory requirements.

The design of the repeat-dose studies allows an opportunity for a geared approach. For the *development* model, as earlier outlined, the work should be conducted to ensure regulatory robustness i.e. two species, usually rat and dog, to full GLP for a minimum of 14 days. Assuming success for the development candidate, many companies will elect to conduct 4-week studies to allow maximum opportunity for smooth progression towards further staged clinical milestones.

In the *investigational* model, however, it is proposed that adequate safety assurance for a single human dose can be given by animal studies of seven days' duration, although this should always be judged on a case by case basis. Human safety must always be the highest priority, but compound availability is a critical factor for initiating the animal studies – restriction of the dosing duration in the animal work can therefore be a resource conserving factor at this early stage.

Other studies

CMC/pharmacy support should be designed to ensure the suitable quality of the test article. This support should be kept to a minimum for an *investigational* compound, whereas appropriate Good Manufacturing Practice (GMP) standards will be essential for the regulatory approval of a submission for a *development* candidate.

Toxicokinetics is a prerequisite both for *investigational* and *development* approaches, although such support may be only minimal in relation to intravenous studies. Distribution studies are undoubtedly appropriate for the *development* model but optional for the *investigational* approach.

Given the limited nature of human exposure being considered in this proposal, antigenicity studies would probably not be required other than in exceptional circumstances (e.g. when the drug-class is immunologically reactive, as is known for some antibacterials).

Other special investigations, such as characterisation of cell receptors (pharmacological or drug metabolising) by *in vitro* studies, should be considered on a case by case basis.

Evaluation

On completion of the *investigational* and/or *development* approach, the interpretation of the data needs to be drawn together in a Safety Assessment Document (SAD), in which contributing 'experts' fully discuss the safety aspects and make appropriate recommendations to the clinical pharmacologists.

Group participants

Chairman:
Dr Jack H Dean
President, Sanofi Research Division
Sanofi Winthrop Inc, USA

Rapporteur:
Dr Michael R Jackson
Director of Medicines Safety Evaluation Division
Glaxo Research & Development Limited, UK

Participants:
Dr Paul Branagan
Medical Director
Eisai Europe Limited, UK

Dr D Bruce Campbell
Director, International Scientific Affairs
Servier Research & Development, UK

Professor Donald S Davies
Professor of Biochemical Pharmacology and
Director of the Department of Clinical Pharmacology
Royal Postgraduate Medical School, UK
CMR Safety Evaluation Advisory Board Member

Professor Anthony D Dayan
Professor of Toxicology, DH Department of Toxicology
St Bartholomew's Hospital Medical College, UK
CMR Safety Evaluation Advisory Board Member

Dr Felix A de la Iglesia
Vice President
Pathology & Experimental Toxicology
Parke-Davis Pharmaceutical Research Division, USA

Professor Lars Ekman
Vice President, Safety Assessment – R & D
Astra AB, Sweden

Dr David S Freestone
Independent Consultant, UK
CMR Safety Evaluation Advisory Board Member

Professor Trevor M Jones
Director General
The Association of the British Pharmaceutical Industry, UK
formerly Main Board Director
The Wellcome Foundation Limited, UK

Dr Diane K Jorkasky
Vice President and Director Clinical Pharmacology, North America
SmithKline Beecham Inc, USA

Dr Hiskias G Keizer
Project Leader, Drug Safety
Solvay Duphar BV, The Netherlands

Dr Bernhard E Matter
Head of Compliance GLP/GCP Auditing
Sandoz Pharma Limited, Switzerland

Dr Takehiko Mori
Manager, Regulatory Affairs
Ono Pharmaceutical Company Limited, Japan

Dr Douglas M Morton
Vice President
Lilly Research Laboratories, USA

Professor Gerhard Schlüter
Head, Department of Toxicology
Bayer AG, Germany

Dr Toshimi Usui
Senior General Manager, R&D Division
Janssen-Kyowa Company Limited, Japan

Dr Herman Van Cauteren
Vice President Nonclinical Safety Assessment
Janssen Research Foundation, Belgium

11 The duration of toxicity studies required to support repeated dosing in humans in clinical investigation

PHILIP BENTLEY and ALAN DUNTON

In attempting to define the requirements for repeat-dose testing in relation to clinical trials, the participants of this discussion group assumed that a certain amount of preclinical data will be available before a new medicine is administered to man for the first time, including absorption, distribution, metabolism and excretion (ADME) data and some genetic toxicology. These preclinical studies will not be discussed further. The design of the repeat-dose toxicity studies is not addressed, but these should be conducted according to current guidelines, in two species with the appropriate toxicokinetic support.

Generally, the approach taken to defining the repeat-dose toxicity testing requirements to support clinical development of a medicine should be as flexible as possible. This proposal is therefore aimed at defining minimal requirements, accepting that there will be cases where considerably more information may be required.

Duration of repeat-dose toxicity studies

It is considered that the duration of repeat-dose studies should be in line with that which the Food and Drug Administration (FDA) presently accepts. For Phase I and Phase II this is a 1:1 relationship between the duration of the toxicity studies and the duration of the clinical study, and in Phase III a 3:1 relationship. This is largely a pragmatic suggestion, but does take into account the design of Phase III trials which have larger patient populations, probably with less control, than Phase I or Phase II trials. In actual fact, if this flexibility can be achieved, it will not have an adverse effect on company strategy because the necessary animal studies are usually available at these stages.

The minimum duration of animal studies should be at least 14 days. This would mean a change in Japan where the guidelines currently recommend a minimum duration of 28 days. However, there will be cases when longer studies are appropriate, and this should be the decision of the company based on the available data. The maximum duration to support clinical trials should be six months. Rather than re-opening the debate of the 12-month dog study, it is proposed that where this study is requested, it should be as a registration requirement rather than one for clinical trials.

Carcinogenicity studies

As the utility of the second rodent species was not discussed, this proposal assumes that two species are routinely used for oncogenicity studies. It was agreed that they should be completed for registration if the intended treatment period exceeds six months. However, there was a division of opinion regarding when these studies should be initiated.

The discussants suggested that carcinogenicity studies should be initiated before starting a clinical trial of six months or longer. This would mean that the animal studies are always ahead of the clinical trial, so before a trial reaches six months, the animals will have been treated for seven or eight months. This is one way of maintaining at least a 1:1 ratio (duration of animal studies: duration of clinical studies) for long-term clinical trials, which many people believe is ethically imperative. The proposal to have a 3:1 ratio in Phase III would not make sense if the animal studies were only six months in duration as Phase III trials may extend to a year or more. An ongoing carcinogenicity study does provide some useful information. Although the finalised data assessment is not available, clinical observations are made throughout and those animals dying spontaneously before the end of the study are autopsied, revealing any serious, unanticipated toxicity.

In discussing this proposal with other participants at the meeting, it became apparent that opinion is divided on this point. A good 6-month animal study will provide a considerable amount of useful data. Furthermore it might not be of value to begin the carcinogenicity study before there is good evidence of efficacy, which may not be obtained in clinical trials with a duration of less than six months. Several toxicologists and clinicians believe that, as the carcinogenicity studies have to be completed before submission for a Product Licence, they should be initiated at the right strategically planned time to ensure that they are not on the critical path, but not for any other reason. Others would like to have some animal studies of longer than six months' exposure when patients are in trial for longer than six months, and the carcinogenicity studies provide an opportunity to obtain such information.

In practice, the proposal to initiate carcinogenicity studies prior to initiating clinical trials of six months or longer should make little difference to most companies. They are almost always started by the time this clinical stage is reached as a delay in initiating carcinogenicity studies can place them on the critical path. Furthermore, there is still a requirement in certain European countries to have the carcinogenicity studies underway before initiating long-term clinical studies.

Presentation of data

Presentation of summary data should be sufficient, at least for Phase I and Phase II. This proposal would require a change in the current FDA requirement for complete study reports. Opinion was divided regarding the presentation of data supporting Phase III clinical trials. Some believe there could be an advantage in submitting full reports for Phase III as it would introduce regulators to the compound before submission of the New Drug Application (NDA), which may help with the NDA review. The recommendation, therefore, addresses only Phase I and II and leaves Phase III open.

Summary

The proposal is summarised in Table 11.1.

Table 11.1 Proposal for duration of studies to support repeat dosing in humans

1.	*Duration of studies*		
	Accept current FDA practice:	Phase I & II	1:1*
		Phase III	3:1*
	Minimum duration to support clinical trials:		14 days
	Maximum duration to support clinical trials:		6 months
2.	*Carcinogenicity studies:*	required if clinical trial duration exceeds 6 months should be initiated before 6-month clinical trials	
3.	*Presentation of data:*	summary reports should be sufficient for Phases I and II	

* Ratio of duration of treatment period in toxicity studies compared to maximal treatment period in clinical trial

Group participants

Chairman:
Dr Alan Dunton
Vice President, Clinical Research and Development
Janssen Research Foundation, USA
formerly Vice President and Director
Center for Clinical Pharmacology and Pharmacokinetics
Syntex (USA) Inc, USA

Rapporteur:
Dr Philip Bentley
Head, Preclinical Safety, Europe
Ciba-Geigy Limited, Switzerland

Participants:
Dr Andrew Aldridge
Manager, Toxicology Projects Group,
Safety of Medicines Department
Zeneca Pharmaceuticals, UK

Dr John C Alexander
Executive Vice President, Medical Research
Searle, USA

Dr Andreas Hofmann
Head of Institute of Toxicology
E Merck, Germany

Dr Toshiji Igarashi
Director, R & D Documentation and Information Technology
Eisai Company Limited, Japan

Dr Harrie FP Joosten
Toxicology Expert
NV Organon, The Netherlands

Professor Laurence J King
Professor of Biochemistry, School of Biological Sciences
University of Surrey, UK
CMR Safety Evaluation Advisory Board Member

Dr Bruce McCullough
Senior Director, General Toxicology
Schering–Plough Research Institute, USA

Dr Wolfgang Neumann
Head, Department of Toxicology
Boehringer Ingelheim KG, Germany

Professor John O'Grady
European Medical Director
Daiichi Pharmaceuticals UK Limited, UK

M David C Scales
Director of Toxicological Sciences
Glaxo Research & Development Limited, UK

Dr Peter L Sibley
Executive Director, Drug Safety Evaluation
Bristol-Myers Squibb Company, USA

Dr J Wilson Totten
Director of Medical & Regulatory Affairs
Fisons plc, UK

12 The timing of reproductive toxicity studies in relation to clinical trials

JEANNE MANSON and FRITZ BÜHLER

Females of childbearing potential (FCBP) (between the ages of 15 and 44) and children (under the age of 18) should be considered for inclusion in early clinical trials of medicines if they constitute a substantial portion of the patient population to be treated. The purpose of inclusion in early trials is to determine whether major differences in safety, pharmacokinetics or pharmacodynamics exist relative to adult male volunteers or females of non-childbearing potential (FNCBP). This information is to be used primarily in the design of subsequent efficacy trials in these populations.

First entry into clinical trials with FCBP and children is not recommended; enrolment of FCBP should occur when safety/tolerability is understood in men or in FNCBP when possible.

The primary responsibility for ensuring that FCBP are not pregnant at the time of enrolment into trials and are monitored for pregnancy induction during the trial resides with the clinician. The high rate of unintentional/unplanned pregnancies in the general population (see Appendix 12.1) underscores the need to provide adequate counselling as well as careful consideration of the type of contraception used (see Appendix 12. 2), and the frequency with which pregnancy tests should be conducted in early clinical trials with FCBP.

Monitoring of serum beta-human chorionic gonadotrophin (β-HCG) constitutes the most sensitive method for early pregnancy detection; elevations in β-HCG can be detected as early as 8–10 days after fertilisation; a urinary β-HCG test can be used in conjunction with the serum test. Decisions on the frequency and type of test (serum or urinary) should be given detailed consideration depending on the length of the trial and what is known about the reproductive toxicity of the agent/pharmaceutical class.

Informed consent of FCBP is particularly important and should contain information concerning foetal and reproductive risk, including any information from reproductive toxicity studies (preliminary or definitive). Information should be sought on the type of contraception used and the patient's consent should be obtained to continue using this method throughout the study period (and later if drug levels persist after termination of treatment). In addition, the consent form should include specific information about pregnancy testing to be done during the trial.

Distinction between escalating single-dose trials versus multiple-dose trials is important in determining the design of trials and identification of essential animal reproductive toxicity studies. As the recommendation is being made that single-/multiple-dose safety/efficacy trials will be completed in males and FNCBP prior to enrolling FCBP, use of terminology such as Phase I, II, etc. is misleading in this context. Phase I trials, in particular, would not be conducted simultaneously in males/FNCBP and FCBP.

1. Single ascending dose trials (up to 7 exposures); multiple-dose trials involving continuous exposure of up to 7 days

Single ascending dose trials are commonly of a design where a single dose is administered followed by a wash-out period. This may be repeated up to seven times but at increasingly higher doses.

Males; females of non-childbearing potential (post-menopausal, hysterectomy, tubal ligation, etc)

Studies required should include genetic toxicity; repeat-dose toxicity studies in two species of appropriate duration with pharmacokinetics and histopathology/organ weights of reproductive organs. There is no perceived need for a male fertility test with a mating trial or with quantitative sperm assessment at this stage.

Females of childbearing potential

A point of debate in this meeting, which was not resolved, was whether females on oral or implanted steroidal contraceptives should be considered as being of childbearing or non-childbearing potential. This is a key point and should be discussed further, since this may determine what studies are required to support this particular stage of clinical development.

Females of childbearing potential should be enrolled only after previous human treatment of males/FNCBP to determine safety/kinetics/pharmacological mode of action. Pregnancy tests and adequate contraception should be used as primary controls to ensure low risk of pregnancy. If there is concern about exposure to this population, greater emphasis should be placed on increased control of clinical trials (more frequent pregnancy tests; more stringent modes of contraception) rather than additional animal studies*. If pregnancy is detected during single ascending dose trials, the female volunteer should be withdrawn from the trial, counselled about the possible sequelae of the exposure, and the outcome of pregnancy monitored to the time of birth as a minimum. Additional monitoring of the new-born should be conducted on a case by case basis, depending on what is known about the reproductive toxicity of the agent/pharmaceutical class.

There was considerable debate about what types of animal studies should be required under these conditions when stringent control is maintained in trials to ensure a low risk of pregnancy. There was general agreement that some type of animal data was necessary to provide adequate information for informed consent and to determine if the agent had a high level of reproductive risk. However, there was no consensus on the specific studies to be performed with recommendations including: no special reproductive toxicity studies carried out; conducting a limited study in a small number of pregnant rats (treatment from gestation day (GD) 6 throughout pregnancy to post-natal day (LD) 20) and rabbits (treatment from GD 7 to 20) and having results but not reports available; conducting definitive embryo/foetal toxicity studies in two species under GLP with full reports available; conducting a female fertility study with treatment for two weeks before mating, throughout mating to the time of implantation (GD 7) followed by a mid-pregnancy Caesarian-section for determining embryo/foetal viability. The latter proposal was considered particularly relevant as pregnancy in human clinical trials would be detected in the post-implantation period, but

---

*Post-meeting note: a review of the literature by J Manson has indicated that even for agents known to have high potency for reducing efficacy of steroidal contraceptives, continuous treatment for several weeks was necessary to induce this effect (Back and Orme, 1990; Szoka and Edgren, 1988). Consequently, this is not likely to be an issue for single ascending dose trials.

pre-implantation exposure could not be monitored nor avoided except through abstention or contraception. If there was concern about prolonged half-life of the test agent, animal studies should include embryo/foetal evaluation in two species. More discussion is needed to resolve these issues. The requirement for animal studies cannot be considered in isolation from the types of controls that will be maintained in the clinic.

Children

The most important criteria for enrolment of children are adequate previous human adult exposure with high expectation of efficacy in children. Children should be enrolled as patients and not as volunteers. Necessary preclinical testing prior to enrolment of children in single ascending dose trials includes a core battery of genetic toxicity tests; repeat-dose toxicity studies in two species of appropriate duration and reproductive toxicity studies with post-natal assessment.

2. Multiple-dose trials involving continuous exposure of greater than 7 but less than 90 days

Unlike the case with single ascending dose trials, there was consensus on the requirements for preclinical studies to enrol FCBP and children in multiple-dose trials of greater than seven days.

Males

This should be the same as above for single ascending dose trials, i.e. repeat-dose toxicity studies in two species of appropriate duration would provide sensitive information on the status of reproductive organs. Given the insensitivity of mating trials, a male fertility study would not yield important information.

Females of non-childbearing potential

This also should be the same as for single ascending dose trials. Treatment in repeat-dose toxicity tests would normally exceed the duration of premating treatment in a female fertility study (two weeks), and would provide sensitive information on the status of reproductive organs.

Females of childbearing potential

The necessary animal studies to enrol FCBP in multiple-dose trials (less than 90 days) would depend on embryo/foetal toxicity studies in two species, a pre-natal/post-natal toxicity study and female fertility study (the full package).

Serum β-HCG tests should be conducted whenever blood samples are drawn, with a consideration of urinary tests at weekly intervals if there was reason for concern. A contraceptive interaction study should be conducted. The potential reduction in contraceptive efficacy of oral/implantable contraceptive steroids by some classes of drugs has been extensively evaluated in the literature. The most common event associated with drugs that reduce contraceptive efficacy is menstrual disturbance, specifically break-through bleeding. It has been claimed that menstrual disturbance may be an early signal of oral contraceptive efficacy failure due to drug interaction. Careful monitoring of signs such as break-through bleeding, amenorrhea and irregular menses may prevent oral contraceptive/drug interactions from resulting in contraceptive failure and unplanned pregnancies (Szoka and Edgren, 1988). It is recommended that women taking contraceptive steroids be carefully evaluated for effects of drug therapy on menstrual disturbance as a primary screen for loss of contraceptive efficacy. Only if disturbances of this type are identified should pharmacokinetic studies on circulating levels of contraceptive steroids be carried out. Such pharmacokinetic studies alone are unlikely to provide reliable information on potential loss of contraceptive efficacy*. As the metabolism of contraceptive steroids is well understood, it is recommended that

*Pharmacokinetic evaluations of circulating contraceptive steroids have not proven to be useful in predicting the potential of concomitant drug therapy to interfere with contraceptive efficacy. Jung-Hoffman and Kuhl (1990) found no correlation between individual ethinylestradiol and progestogen levels and the occurrence of intermenstrual bleeding in women evaluated across 12 cycles of treatment. This was due to large intra-individual and inter-individual variations in the serum levels of the contraceptive steroids. Orme (1982) found a 20- to 30-fold variation in the steady state plasma concentrations of ethinylestradiol and levonorgesterol in women on oral contraceptive therapy. This was believed to be due to a large first pass effect from highly variable sulphate conjugation in the gut wall. Guengerich (1990) considers the high variability in circulating contraceptive steroid levels is due to variations in the levels of liver and gut cytochrome P450 IIIA4, the major catalyst of the 2-hydroxylation reaction of ethinylestradiol.

preclinical models be utilised to predict which agents have the potential to reduce steroidal contraceptive efficacy in humans.

Children

There were arguments for and against consideration being given to doing a juvenile toxicity study in a non-rodent species (dog or primate) with appropriately aged animals relative to children enrolled in trials. The availability of the necessary scientific expertise in conducting and interpreting these studies was considered by some to be limited, whereas others believed that there were circumstances where such studies provided valuable information.

3. Multiple-dose trials, continuous exposure greater than 90 days (including marketing application)

Males; females of non-childbearing potential

In addition to the recommendations for studies to support clinical trials of up to 90 days, investigations should include a male fertility study to support enrolment of males.

Females of childbearing potential

Investigations should include serum β-HCG test before the first treatment and after the last treatment to provide adequate follow-up should pregnancy occur. Optimum contraceptive use should continue from single-dose studies. When pregnancies occur in trials despite these precautions, the patient should be discontinued from the protocol, treatment may be continued if the benefit clearly outweighs the risk. Patients should be counselled and pregnancy outcome monitored to the time of birth as a minimum.

Post-marketing surveillance (PMS) for effects of drugs on pregnancy is important and should be strengthened. There is therefore a need to find a good international database for PMS of drug exposure during pregnancy and effects on pregnancy outcome (Pincott, 1994).

Summary

A summary of this proposal for the timing of reproductive toxicity studies in relation to clinical trials is presented in Table 12.1.

Table 12.1 Proposal for the timing of reproductive toxicity studies in relation to clinical trials

Clinical population	*Clinical considerations*	*Reproductive toxicity studies to support clinical phase*		
		Single ascending dose trials (up to 7 exposures) and multiple-dose up to 7 days	*Multiple-dose trials, continuous exposure of greater than 7 and less than 90 days*	*Multiple-dose trials, continuous exposure of greater than 90 days*
Males	Initial population for clinical study	Genetic toxicology. Repeat-dose studies with pharmacokinetics and histopathology/ organ weights of reproductive organs	No additional recommendations	As before plus male fertility study
Females of non-child-bearing potential (FNCBP)	Initial population for clinical study	Genetic toxicology. Repeat-dose studies with pharmacokinetics and histopathology/ organ weights of reproductive organs.	No additional recommendations	No additional recommendations
Females of childbearing potential (FCBP)	Enrol after previous treatment of males or FNCBP. Use of pregnancy testing and adequate contraceptive cover	No consensus reached on exact studies. Further discussion required.	Female fertility study. Embryo/foetal developmental toxicity study in two species. Pre- and post-natal developmental toxicity study. Oral contraceptive interaction study	No additional recommendations
Children	Use patients only, high expectation of efficacy. Enrol when previous adult human exposure data is available	As for males/FNCBP plus reproductive toxicity studies including post-natal assessment	Consideration given to conducting a juvenile toxicity study in a non-rodent species on a case by case basis	No additional recommendations

References

Back DJ and Orme ML'E (1990). Pharmacokinetic drug interactions with oral contraceptives. *Clinical Pharmocokinetics* **18(6)**:472–484.

Forrest JD and Singh S (1990). The sexual and reproductive behavior of American women, 1982–1988. *Family Planning Perspectives* **22 (5)**: 206.

Guengerich FP (1990). Metabolism of 17a-ethinylestradiol in humans. *Life Sciences* **47**: 1981–1988.

Jones EF and Forrest JD (1992). Contraceptive failure rates based on the 1988 NSFG. *Family Planning Perspectives* **24 (1)**: 12–19.

Jung-Hoffman C and Kuhl H (1990). Pharmacokinetics and pharmacodynamics of oral contraceptive steroids: Factors influencing steroid metabolism. *American Journal of Obstetrics and Gynecology* **163**: 83–97.

Orme ML'E (1982). The clinical pharmacology of oral contraceptive steroids. *British Journal of Clinical Pharmacology* **14**: 31–42.

Pincott J (1994). *Oral communication:* Reproductive and developmental toxicity studies required to support the inclusion of women and children in clinical trials. CMR Discussion Meeting on The Timing of Toxicological Studies to Support Clinical Trials, Nutfield Priory, Surrey, England. May 9th & 10th 1994.

Szoka PR and Edgren RA (1988). Drug interactions with oral contraceptives: Compilation and analysis of an adverse experience report database. *Fertility and Sterility* **49 (5)**: 31S–38S.

Appendix 12.1 Estimated outcome of unintentional pregnancies in women aged 15–44 years in the USA (adapted from Forrest and Singh, 1990)

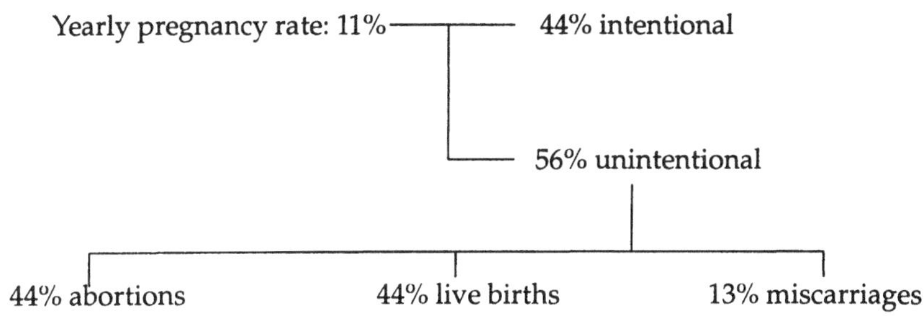

Appendix 12.2 Failure rates of methods of contraception in the USA (adapted from Jones and Forrest, 1992)

Method of contraception	*Failure rate*
Oral contraceptive pill	8%
Condom	15%
Spermicides	26%
Periodic abstinence	26%

N.B. Failure rates vary more by user characteristics such as age, marital status and economic status than by method, suggesting that contraceptive failure results more from improper and irregular use rather than from the inherent limitations of the method.

Group participants

Chairman:
Professor Fritz R Bühler
Director, International Clinical Research
Hoffmann-La Roche Limited, Switzerland

Rapporteur:
Dr Jeanne M Manson
Distinguished Senior Investigator
Merck Research Laboratories, USA

Participants:
Dr Frank M Armstrong
Head of Medical Research Department
Zeneca Pharmaceuticals, UK

Dr Gerd Bode
Head, Toxicology, Safety & Molecular
Roussel Uclaf, France

Dr Ian Gaunt
Head of Toxicology, UK
SmithKline Beecham Pharmaceuticals, UK

Professor Robert Hess
Consultant in Toxicology and Pathology, Switzerland
CMR Safety Evaluation Advisory Board Member

Dr Yasumoto Kikuchi
Consultant, Asia/Pacific Division
Procter & Gamble, Japan

Mr David Kinch
Director of Toxicology
Syntex Research Centre, UK

Dr Alastair M Monro
Director, External Scientific Affairs
Central Research Divison, Pfizer Inc, USA

Dr Hugh E Morgan
Head of Toxicology
Boots Pharmaceuticals, UK

Dr John R Pincott
Medical Director, European Safety Assurance, Regulatory Affairs
Pfizer Inc, UK

Dr Kurt E Suter
Head of Project Group, Toxicology Department of Drug Safety
Sandoz Pharma Limited, Switzerland

Dr Edward T Yau
Executive Director of Toxicology
Ciba-Geigy Corporation, USA

Dr Robert L Zerbe
Senior Vice President, Worldwide Clinical Investigation
Parke-Davis Pharmaceutical Research, USA

13 The way forward

GWYN MORGAN

Summary

1. Under the auspices of the International Conference of Harmonisation (ICH), significant progress has been made toward harmonising practices and procedures in certain areas of toxicology. While the focus of earlier ICH topics was mainly concerned with achieving scientific and technical harmonisation, agreement on the timing of toxicity studies in relation to clinical trials will have a direct impact on the process of drug development.

2. In adopting harmonised guidelines on toxicity testing, primary consideration must be given to: (i) the quality of the toxicological data; (ii) the relevance of the data in relation to the objectives of the proposed clinical trials; and (iii) the interpretation of the data in the context of risk versus benefit to the patient.

3. Harmonisation should be seen clearly as a joint initiative by government regulatory agencies and the pharmaceutical industry to rationalise the cost of drug development in order to increase the availability of new medicines while, at the same time, ensuring that proper standards of drug safety are upheld.

Introduction

The International Conference on Harmonisation (ICH), now in its third epoch, has done much to focus attention on the disparities which exist in the regulatory practices and policies of the three major regions (the USA, Japan and Europe) in which government-funded agencies regulate the development of new pharmaceutical entities and the marketing of pharmaceutical products. Significant progress has been made toward harmonising practices and procedures in certain areas of toxicology. For example, the new tripartite guideline for the evaluation of new compounds in reproductive toxicology, is a significant advance. Consensus is currently being sought in the discussions on other topics, such as genetic toxicology and various aspects of carcinogenicity assessment, in preparation for the Third International Conference on Harmonisation (ICH3), to be held in Yokohama, Japan, in November 1995. While the focus of earlier ICH topics was mainly concerned with achieving scientific and technical harmonisation which has since influenced the design and conduct of toxicology studies, the topic reviewed at this meeting will have a direct impact on the process of drug development and the manner in which it will be regulated globally. Moreover, consideration of issues related to the timing (and duration) of toxicity studies required to support clinical studies, unlike the technical focus of earlier ICH topics, takes us beyond the boundaries of toxicology as a scientific discipline into the realm of public debate. Though the issues are more complex, it is evident from the discussion that took place at this meeting that an opportunity exists to devise regulatory policies and strategies that extend considerably beyond a formulaic approach to drug development. Indeed, a codified set of rules to be adopted as a universal guideline under the rubric of harmonisation may not be the most desirable outcome of future deliberations on this topic. A number of constituencies will be engaged in, and affected by, the effort to harmonise toxicological study requirements in support of clinical trials. As always, the safety of human patients is paramount, but the future of drug development on a national, as well as international, scale is also very much at issue. If industrial and regulatory scientists seize the initiative to think afresh about the process of drug development, they will recognise opportunities to establish a consensus that will enable us, in future, to adopt a more flexible, case by case approach to the regulatory approval of clinical development programmes. While it may not be perceived to be in the interest of public safety if we adopt the least demanding of the regional requirements for toxicity studies in support of clinical trials worldwide, it could be detrimental to the public interest, and the advancement of medicine, if we adopt the most conservative of the regional requirements.

Also to be considered is the urgent need for new medical treatment in certain diseases, the cost of drug development, the impact of regulations on the cost of drugs, and the potential pharmacoeconomic benefit to the global community.

The contribution of toxicology

There are many inconsistencies and irregularities between the existing requirements for toxicity studies to support clinical trials in the three regulatory regions. This incongruity between the regions as regards their implementation of regulatory policy must also reflect differences in their perception of toxicological data and the utility of those data in governing the design and duration of clinical trials. The first step in harmonisation should be a clear understanding of the purpose and limitations of toxicology data. The role of toxicology in drug development is often misunderstood and the expectations of toxicological data are frequently misplaced. Toxicology is frequently cited for failing to predict the occurrence of adverse events in humans. This charge is obviously difficult to prove or refute, since the principal objective of toxicology is to prevent exposure of humans to toxic chemicals in the first place. Besides, toxicological data should preclude exposure of humans to dosages of a new drug that proved to be toxic in animals. Indeed, it may be said, with relief, that it is the human species which fails to validate many of the toxic effects observed in animals. The principal objective of toxicological studies should be to characterise the toxic effects of investigational drugs in a manner that is relevant to their intended use in clinical trials. As such, toxicological studies should be viewed as surrogates of subsequent clinical trials. Exposure to the drug must be well defined in terms of its absorption, distribution, metabolism and excretion. Appropriate endpoints must be measured to ensure detection and accurate quantification of the toxic effects evoked. Finally, the relationships between dose, exposure and effect must be interpreted in a context that is relevant to the planned clinical trials. Interpretation of toxicological data (in the context of risk to the patient versus clinical benefit) is the most vital element in the communication between the toxicologist, the clinician and the reviewer in a regulatory agency. For most drugs and chemicals investigated in toxicology, the manifestation of toxicity is determined to varying degrees by the dose administered and the duration of exposure. However, in the absence of appropriate dose selection and measurement of relevant endpoints, it is unlikely that extending the duration of a toxicity study will ensure the complete characterisation of a drug's toxic potential. In other words, mandating the duration of toxicity studies in an empirical fashion according to the length of a proposed clinical trial does not make a significant contribution to the process of risk/benefit analysis if these other scientific objectives have not been met by the design and execution of the supporting toxicity studies. It is important, therefore, that the adoption and implementation of harmonised guidelines should give primary consideration to: (i) the quality of the toxicological data generated; (ii) the relevance of the data in relation to the objectives of the proposed clinical trials; and (iii) the interpretation of the data in the context of risk versus benefit afforded to the patient. If toxicologists, clinicians and reviewers in regulatory agencies focus on these three essential elements in applications to conduct clinical trials on a compound by compound basis, and seek a common understanding of the issues, then the process of drug development will be greatly improved.

The public perception of drug regulation

The effort to harmonise guidelines and introduce consistency into toxicological study requirements in support of clinical trials can yield many significant benefits. It is commonplace for clinical development programmes to cross national ethnic and cultural boundaries. This multinational approach improves global access to new therapies and ensures that the safety of new drugs is evaluated from diverse vantage points. The economic well-being of the pharmaceutical industry and the safety and health of the world population are well served by clinical development programmes of this global scale. It is both timely and logical, therefore, to re-examine the current requirements for toxicity studies in support of clinical trials in order to bring international guidelines into line with the scope and scale of clinical development programmes. However, harmonisation must not be perceived by the public or any other agency (claiming to advocate public safety in any quarter of the world) as a means of introducing less rigorous standards for the safety of medicines. Rather, it should be seen as a joint initiative by government regulatory agencies and the pharmaceutical industry to rationalise the cost of drug development in order to increase the availability of new medicines while, at the same time, ensuring that proper standards are upheld to sustain the safety of drugs. Again, communication of these ideals and goals should be a joint responsibility of regulatory agencies and pharmaceutical companies. The safety of drugs is an issue which is very much in the public domain. Unfortunately, reports of adverse events are more often purveyed by the public media than are the therapeutic and economic gains enjoyed by society at large as a result of costly and innovative research and development carried out by the pharmaceutical industry. It is important that we, the pharmaceutical industry, and our peers in governmental agencies, articulate these goals of harmonisation to the public at large in order to ensure that this co-operative effort is perceived as a gain to society without infringing ethical or scientific standards which must be upheld to assure the safety of medicines in the future.

Conclusion

This meeting has been a useful discussion forum on a most important aspect of drug development. The proceedings of this meeting have been published as points to consider in the discussions that will take place under the auspices of ICH, involving other industrial colleagues as well as representatives from academia and governmental regulatory agencies. This meeting has fulfilled its purpose in preparing for a more effective discussion in the forum of ICH, and the ultimate product of this endeavour will be presented for general review at ICH3.

14 Input to ICH

R MICHAEL McCLAIN

Summary

1. The overall objective of the International Conference on Harmonisation (ICH) process is to expedite drug development and increase the availability of new medicines to patients. Within the area of safety evaluation, activities focus on harmonising and improving guidelines/regulations in order to achieve the mutual acceptance of toxicological data and to eliminate redundant testing. The timing of toxicity studies in relation to clinical investigation was adopted as a topic for discussion at the ICH Steering Committee Meeting in March 1994. This will be a joint effort of the Safety and Efficacy Working Parties.

2. The main regional differences in existing guidelines are the requirement for a fertility study prior to Phase I in Japan, the 6-month chronic toxicity study that is required for clinical trials longer than one month in the EC and Japan, the need for final study reports in the USA, the timing of carcinogenicity studies and of reproductive toxicity studies to support the inclusion of women in clinical trials. Discussions on these issues have already begun and some progress has been made to resolving the differences.

3. The ICH guideline on the timing of toxicity studies is still very much in the formative stage and the input from these proceedings will be useful during the progress towards international harmonisation. A carefully balanced degree of flexibility within the new guideline should allow toxicological evaluations to be conducted in a manner appropriate for each particular compound.

ICH procedures

The International Conference on Harmonisation (ICH) was established to serve primarily as a forum for discussion between regulatory and industry scientists from the three major geographic regions, namely Europe, Japan and the USA. The main purpose with regard to safety testing is to harmonise the guidelines/regulations in order to achieve the mutual acceptance of toxicological data and to eliminate redundant testing. The overall objective of the ICH process is to expedite the drug development process and hasten the availability of new medicines for therapeutic use. The timing of toxicity studies in relation to clinical investigation was adopted as a Safety and Efficacy topic at the ICH Steering Committee Meeting in March 1994. It is still at a very early stage, so the input from this meeting will be very useful as this topic proceeds through the different stages.

Topics for discussion within the ICH process are selected by the ICH Steering Committee on the advice of the Expert Working Groups. Once a topic has been agreed, the discussions proceed through five steps (Table 14.1). At Step One, a preliminary discussion of the topic is held by the Expert Working Group (EWG). The objective of this discussion is for the regulatory and industry representatives to reach a consensus on the major issues. Currently, the timing issue is at Step One and the EWG is in the process of preparing the preliminary draft of the Step One paper. Once a consensus draft is reached by the Expert Working Group, it is sent to the Steering Committee, and it is hoped that such a draft on Timing will be ready for presentation to the Steering Committee in October 1994. At Step Two this consensus draft is sent to the regulatory agencies who circulate it for comment by the public, industry and others. The period for comment is usually six months. At Step Three, the comments are taken into consideration and the final draft is prepared. This is then signed off by the Expert Working Group. At Step Four, the Steering Committee endorses the final draft and recommends its adoption as a tripartite guideline. Finally, at Step Five the regulatory agencies in the various regions change their regulations and guidelines in order to incorporate the agreed tripartite guideline. The goal for Timing is to reach Step 4 by ICH3 in November 1995.

There is substantial industry involvement in Steps One and Two, and some at Step Three to the extent that industry representatives sign off the draft. However, by the time Steps Four and Five are

Table 14.1 The ICH process

STEP 1	
	Preliminary Discussions of topic by EWG Preliminary Draft (guideline, policy statement, recommendation, points to consider) Consensus Draft to Steering Committee
STEP 2	
	Consensus Draft to Regulatory Agencies and Others for formal consultation (comment period - 6 months)
STEP 3	
	Comments collected and exchanged by Regulatory Agencies and Others Regulatory Rapporteur amends Draft Sign off by EWG
STEP 4	
	Steering Committee endorses Final Draft and recommends adoption
STEP 5	
	Recommendations incorporated into domestic regulations

reached, the final decisions are in the hands of the regulatory agencies, although there is still the opportunity for discussion and input. The initial Steps are therefore important, since the final guideline reflects both the regulatory and industry input. Many regulators see this as a positive factor of the ICH process, in that they are now obtaining a perspective from experienced industry scientists, that they otherwise would not have obtained. Each step of drug development is examined from the viewpoint of, 'is it really necessary, can we do it differently, can we do it better?'. This is probably the reason why the ICH process has been so effective and is able to achieve the goal of expediting and improving the process rather than hindering things and resulting in unnecessary work.

The Steering Committee and the Expert Working Groups within Quality, Safety and Efficacy are comprised of one person from each of the regulatory regions and a representative from each of the regional pharmaceutical manufacturers' associations. The members of the EWG on timing of toxicity studies are shown in Table 14.2.

Table 14.2 Expert Working Group* on timing of toxicity studies

Dr M Burns	Commission of the European Community (CEC)	Dr M McClain *Roche (Rapporteur)*	Pharmaceutical Research and Manufacturers of America (PhRMA)
Dr J Cavagnaro Dr A Taylor	US Food and Drug Administration (FDA)	Dr D Scales, *Glaxo* Dr P Lehnar, *Sanofi*	European Federation of Pharmaceutical Industries' Associations (EFPIA)
Mr K Misawa Dr Y Hayashi,	Japanese Ministry of Health and Welfare (MHW)	Dr Hiroshi, *Takeda*	Japan Pharmaceutical Manufacturers Association (JPMA)

*This topic is a joint effort for Safety and Efficacy. The EWG for Efficacy to be appointed.

Major issues with regard to timing

The major regional differences in the existing guidelines on timing have been covered in the chapter by Scales and Usui in this publication. Basically, the main differences are the requirement for the fertility study prior to Phase I in Japan, the 6-month chronic toxicity study that is required for clinical trials in excess of one month in the EC and Japan, the need for final study reports, particularly to open the investigational new drug (IND) which is a more stringent requirement in the USA and the issue of the carcinogenicity studies

Table 14.3 Regional differences

1.	Male fertility study prior to Phase I	– Japan
2.	Six-month chronic toxicity for trials of more than one month duration	– Japan, Europe
3.	Final study reports	– USA
4.	Carcinogenicity studies	– USA >3 months – EC >6 months

(Table 14.3). In addition, one of the most difficult issues we have to deal with is the inclusion of women in clinical trials. These topics were all discussed at the meeting of the Expert Working Group in Tokyo, in March 1994.

Male fertility study

There was considerable discussion at this meeting in March 1994, on the male fertility study. A presentation was made on the collaborative effort between the JPMA and the MHW which showed that male fertility studies do not provide much useful information One can gain all the information that is necessary, at least for early clinical trials, based on good histopathology of the testes and a two-week evaluation would be sufficient. The Japanese may therefore be willing to eliminate the requirement for male fertility testing prior to an introduction in Phase I clinical trials.

Six-month chronic toxicity study

With respect to the requirement for a 6-month chronic toxicity study for clinical trials in excess of one month, the Japanese and EC representatives discussed a recommendation to move to the US standard which, in general terms, would be that the duration of the clinical studies can be equal to the duration of the toxicity studies. US-based companies have been doing clinical trials for more than 30 years to the current US Food and Drug Administration (FDA) standards. There appears to be nothing wrong with the way these clinical trials are conducted and there have been no major problems. It is considered, therefore, that it is not necessary to go beyond the US standards.

Final study reports

Opening the IND in the USA requires more time because of the need for final study reports. There is some discussion with the FDA about accepting draft reports, although no recommendations have been made. The EWG is aware that delays may encourage companies to do studies in other regions, thus this is under discussion. In practice, the chronic study final reports are not necessary to continue clinical trials. Ongoing chronic studies would support the continuation of clinical trials with the provision of summary reports and, of course, if a significant adverse finding was identified it would have to be reported.

Carcinogenicity studies

The FDA has maintained that carcinogenicity studies are necessary if the clinical treatment is over three months and the EU maintains that it is necessary only if treatment is in excess of six months. This issue is not resolved. Within the EU, the Committee for Proprietary Medicinal Products (CPMP) Safety Working Party is reluctant to change the six-month requirement without a scientific justification and the FDA has problems in changing its requirement from three to six months. An agreement of three months may actually be of benefit to the industry, because in the USA the only guideline published in the Federal Register refers to six weeks clinical use as invoking the requirement for carcinogenicity studies. A compromise that has been suggested is that if a three-month standard is adopted, this would only relate to continuous treatment. However, if the six-month standard were accepted, this would probably relate to intermittent (accumulated lifetime exposure) as opposed to continuous exposure.

Inclusion of women in clinical trials

One of the more difficult issues that must be dealt with is the inclusion of women in clinical trials. The USA (changes currently under discussion) and Japan require the female part of the fertility test and the teratology studies to be completed prior to the inclusion of women of childbearing potential (WCBP) in clinical trials. Although the USA is currently discussing a change in this restriction, the level of concern for the unintentional exposure of an embryo/foetus in early clinical trials remains unchanged. The EWG agreed that, based upon certain inclusion criteria, women could be safely enrolled in carefully controlled clinical trials prior to the conduct of reproductive toxicity studies. As in the past, the inclusion of women considered not of childbearing potential (postmenopausal, surgically altered (hysterectomy, tubal ligation), etc) could be included.

It was felt that the WCBP could be separated into two categories. First, WCBP on effective birth control, in conjunction with pregnancy testing and informed consent, could be safely included in early clinical trials with a short treatment duration (1–7 days) or short systemic exposure. However, a second category of WCBP, for which control of pregnancy or pregnancy status is unknown, could not be enrolled until the female reproductive toxicity and teratology studies are performed. The consensus of the EWG was that there was no basis to change the level of concern or the requirements in regard to the unintentional exposure of an embryo/foetus prior to an assessment of the potential risks for such an exposure.

Flexibility

Rather than describing the elements of the guidelines as 'minimal requirements', the term 'sufficient requirements' is preferable. In other words, if one does this type of study, this should be sufficient to support the clinical trials. With respect to flexibility, there will be an explicit statement in the guideline. Basically, if the recommendation or guideline fits the situation then it should be utilised. However, each drug is different. What one does in the toxicological evaluation for a compound should be that which is appropriate for that particular compound. Alternative approaches may, however, require an increased amount of discussion and consultation with the regulatory agencies. Flexibility goes two ways. Excessive rigidity in guidelines can result in inappropriate or irrelevant toxicology. On the other hand, too much flexibility or no guidelines at all can result in arbitrary development and protracted debates on the adequacy of a submission. Thus, there needs to be a good balance concerning the flexibility of requirements.

Conclusion

The Expert Working Group has discussed recommendations for harmonisation. It would be premature, however, to conclude that any regulations have changed or will change. It must be borne in mind that we are only at Step One in this process and that there is still a long way go. Recommendations will be further discussed by the Safety and Efficacy groups and changed in due course. The information presented at this meeting will be helpful as these guidelines are modified during the process of harmonisation.

Meeting participants

EUROPE

Dr Andrew Aldridge
Manager, Toxicology Projects Group
Safety of Medicines Department
Zeneca Pharmaceuticals, UK

Dr Frank M Armstrong
Head of Medical Research Department
Zeneca Pharmaceuticals, UK

Dr Philip Bentley
Head, Preclinical Safety, Europe
Ciba-Geigy Limited, Switzerland

Dr Gerd Bode
Head, Toxicology, Safety & Molecular
Roussel Uclaf, France

Dr Paul Branagan
Medical Director
Eisai Europe Limited, UK

Professor Fritz R Bühler
Director, International Clinical Research
Hoffmann-La Roche Limited, Switzerland

Dr D Bruce Campbell
Director, International Scientific Affairs
Servier Research & Development, UK

Professor Donald S Davies
Professor of Biochemical Pharmacology and
Director of the Department of Clinical Pharmacology
Royal Postgraduate Medical School, UK
CMR Safety Evaluation Advisory Board Member

Professor Anthony D Dayan
Professor of Toxicology, DH Department of Toxicology
St Bartholomew's Hospital Medical College, UK
CMR Safety Evaluation Advisory Board Member

Professor Lars Ekman
Vice President, Safety Assessment – R & D
Astra AB, Sweden

Dr David S Freestone
Independent Consultant, UK
CMR Safety Evaluation Advisory Board Member

Dr Ian Gaunt
Head of Toxicology, UK
SmithKline Beecham Pharmaceuticals, UK

Professor Robert Hess
Consultant in Toxicology and Pathology, Switzerland
CMR Safety Evaluation Advisory Board Member

Dr Andreas Hofmann
Head of Institute of Toxicology
E Merck, Germany

Dr Michael R Jackson
Director of Medicines Safety Evaluation Division
Glaxo Research & Development Limited, UK

Professor Trevor M Jones
Director General
The Association of the British Pharmaceutical Industry, UK
formerly Main Board Director
The Wellcome Foundation Limited, UK

Dr Harrie FP Joosten
Toxicology Expert
NV Organon, The Netherlands

Dr Hiskias G Keizer
Project Leader, Drug Safety
Solvay Duphar BV, The Netherlands

Mr David Kinch
Director of Toxicology
Syntex Research Centre, UK

Professor Laurence J King
Professor of Biochemistry, School of Biological Sciences
University of Surrey, UK
CMR Safety Evaluation Advisory Board Member

Dr Cyndy E Lumley
Associate Director
Centre for Medicines Research, UK

Dr Bernhard E Matter
Head of Compliance GLP/GCP Auditing
Sandoz Pharma Limited, Switzerland

Dr Neil McAuslane
Project Manager
Centre for Medicines Research, UK

Dr Hugh E Morgan
Head of Toxicology
Boots Pharmaceuticals, UK

Dr Wolfgang Neumann
Head, Department of Toxicology
Boehringer Ingelheim KG, Germany

Professor John O'Grady
European Medical Director
Daiichi Pharmaceuticals UK Limited, UK

Dr Christopher Parkinson
Senior Research Associate
Centre for Medicines Research, UK

Dr John R Pincott
Medical Director, European Safety Assurance, Regulatory Affairs
Pfizer Inc, UK

M David C Scales
Director of Toxicological Sciences
Glaxo Research & Development Limited, UK

Professor Gerhard Schlüter
Head, Department of Toxicology
Bayer AG, Germany

Dr Kurt E Suter
Head of Project Group, Toxicology Department of Drug Safety
Sandoz Pharma Limited, Switzerland

Dr J Wilson Totten
Director of Medical & Regulatory Affairs
Fisons plc, UK

Dr Herman Van Cauteren
Vice President, Nonclinical Safety Assessment
Janssen Research Foundation, Belgium

Professor Stuart R Walker
Director
Centre for Medicines Research, UK

JAPAN

Dr Toshiji Igarashi
Director, R & D Documentation and Information Technology
Eisai Company Limited, Japan

Dr Yasumoto Kikuchi
Consultant, Asia/Pacific Division
Procter & Gamble, Japan

Dr Takehiko Mori
Manager, Regulatory Affairs
Ono Pharmaceutical Company Limited, Japan

Dr Toshimi Usui
Senior General Manager, Nonclinical Safety Assessment,
R&D Division
Janssen-Kyowa Company Limited, Japan

USA

Dr John C Alexander
Executive Vice President, Medical Research
Searle, USA

Dr Jack H Dean
President, Sanofi Research Divisiont
Sanofi Winthrop Inc, USA

Dr Felix A de la Iglesia
Vice President, Pathology & Experimental Toxicology
Parke-Davis Pharmaceutical Research Division, USA

Dr Alan Dunton
Vice President, Clinical Research and Development
Jannsen Research Foundation, USA
formerly Vice President and Director
Center for Cinical Pharmacology and Pharmacokinetics
Syntex (USA) Inc, USA

Dr Diane K Jorkasky
Vice President and Director Clinical Pharmacology, North America
SmithKline Beecham Inc, USA

Dr Jeanne M Manson
Distinguished Senior Investigator
Merck Research Laboratories, USA

Dr R Michael McClain
Director of Toxicology/Research Advisor
Hoffmann-La Roche Inc, USA

Dr Bruce McCullough
Senior Director, General Toxicology
Schering–Plough Research Institute, USA

Dr Alastair M Monro
Director, External Scientific Affairs
Central Research Divison, Pfizer Inc, USA

Dr Gwyn Morgan
Vice President, Safety Assessment
Research and Development Division
SmithKline Beecham Pharmaceuticals, USA

Dr Douglas M Morton
Vice President
Lilly Research Laboratories, USA

Dr Peter L Sibley
Executive Director, Drug Safety Evaluation
Bristol-Myers Squibb Company, USA

Dr Edward T Yau
Executive Director of Toxicology
Ciba-Geigy Corporation, USA

Dr Robert L Zerbe
Senior Vice President, Worldwide Clinical Investigation
Parke-Davis Pharmaceutical Research, USA

Glossary

ADME	Absorption, distribution, metabolism and excretion
AIDS	Acquired immmune deficiency syndrome
ALT	Alanine transaminase
AST	Aspartate transaminase
AUC	Area under the curve
CEC	Commission of the European Community
CMC	Chemistry manufacturing controls
CNS	Central nervous system
CPMP	Committee for Proprietary Medicinal Products
CVS	Cardiovascular system
EFPIA	European Federation of Pharmaceutical Industries' Associations
EU	European Union (European Community)
EWG	Expert Working Group (of the ICH)
FCBP	Females of childbearing potential
FDA	Food and Drug Administration (USA)
FNCBP	Females of non-childbearing potential
GLP	Good laboratory practice
GMP	Good manufacturing practice
γ-GT	Gamma-glutamyl transferase
β-HCG	Beta-human chorionic gonadotrophin
HTLV-I	Human T-cell leukaemia virus-I
ICH	International Conference on Harmonisation
IND	Investigational new drug
JPMA	Japan Pharmaceutical Manufacturers' Association
LAP	Leucine aminopeptidase
LDH	Lactate dehydrogenase
MAL 4	Medicines Act Leaflet No. 4
MCA	Medicines Control Agency
MHW	Japanese Ministry of Health and Welfare
MPA	Medicinal Products Agency
MTD	Maximum tolerated dose
NDA	New drug application
NDAB	National Drugs Advisory Board
NOEL	No observed effect level
NSAID	Non-steroidal anti-inflammatory drug
PhRMA	Pharmaceutical Research and Manufacturers of America (formerly PMA)
PMA	Pharmaceutical Manufacturers' Association
SAD	Safety assessment document
TAC	Test article characterisation
WCBP	Women of childbearing potential

Index

SPRINGER NATURE

GPSR Compliance

The European Union's (EU) General Product Safety Regulation (GPSR) is a set of rules that requires consumer products to be safe and our obligations to ensure this.

If you have any concerns about our products, you can contact us on ProductSafety@springernature.com

In case Publisher is established outside the EU, the EU authorized representative is:

Springer Nature Customer Service Center GmbH
Europaplatz 3
69115 Heidelberg, Germany

Kolibri 360 GmbH
Ferdinand-Jühlke-Straße 7
99095 Erfurt, Deutschland
produktsicherheit@kolibri360.de